S0-BQM-237

Tumor Markers
Clinical and Laboratory Studies

Tumor Markers
Clinical and Laboratory Studies

Janis V. Klavins, MD, PhD

Professor of Pathology
Cornell University Medical College
New York, New York
Chairman, Department of Pathology
Catholic Medical Center of
Brooklyn and Queens
Jamaica, New York

ALAN R. LISS INC., NEW YORK

Address all Inquiries to the Publisher
Alan R. Liss, Inc., 41 East 11th Street, New York, NY 10003

Printed in the United States of America.

Library of Congress Cataloging in Publication Data

Klavins, Janis V.
Tumor markers.

Bibliography: p.
Includes index.
1. Tumor markers—Diagnostic use. 2. Carcinoembryonic antigens—Diagnostic use. 3. Cancer—Diagnosis.
I. Title. [DNLM: 1. Antigens, Neoplasms—analysis.
QW 573 K63t]
RC270.K55 1985 616.99′4075 85-6799
ISBN 0-8451-0248-6

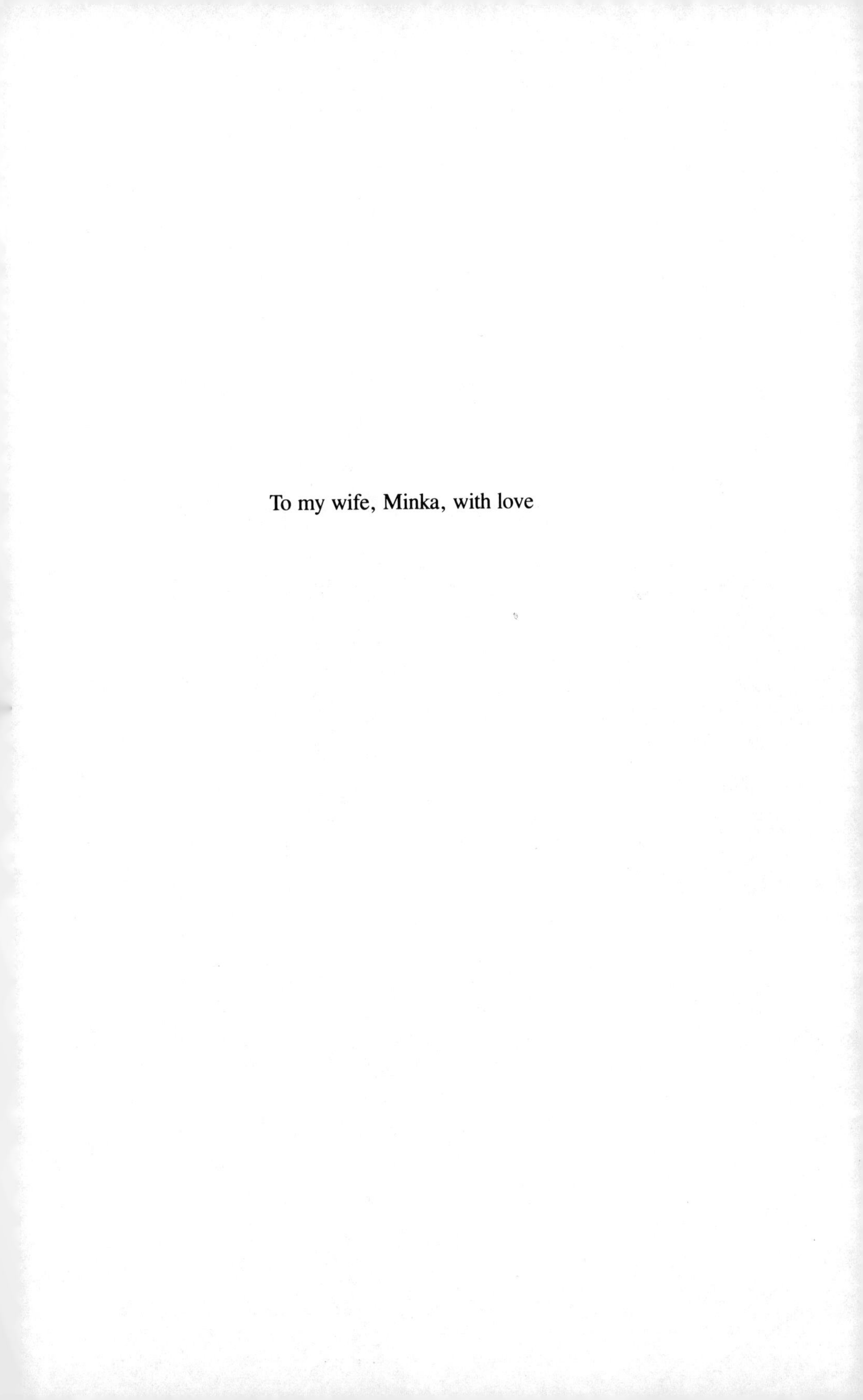

To my wife, Minka, with love

Contents

Preface

This book is intended for clinicians, investigators, and students.

It provides the clinician with a review of the array of tumor markers from which to select the ones most appropriate for follow-up of patients with various forms of malignant neoplasms.

For the investigator it identifies those substances that are potentially specific markers but require additional study to establish their actual value. I have designated many markers as tumor-specific on the basis of preliminary reports that they have not been detected in fetal or non-neoplastic adult tissues. These substances must be subjected to further investigation.

The student will find here an introduction to the various types of tumor markers and to the evidence upon which markers are classified as oncofetal, tumor-associated, or tumor-specific.

Sincere thanks to my family, to my wife, Minka, for her unselfish support and to my children—Ilze, Janis, and especially Lize for drawing the diagrams and Filip for producing some portions of the manuscript.

I am grateful to Sister Regina Clare Woods, Chief Librarian of the Catholic Medical Center of Brooklyn and Queens, and her staff for their outstanding library services. I am especially grateful to Miss Trudy Horowitz for her extraordinary effort to produce the manuscript.

Janis V. Klavins

Introduction

The term *tumor* has been used to designate malignant neoplasms. Malignant neoplasms characteristically develop locally, invade adjacent tissues, spread to various sites of the organism, constitute unpredictable forms, and destroy normally functioning tissue. The term *tumor markers* has been used to designate biological substances that are produced uniquely or in excessive amounts by malignant neoplasms.

The term *tumor* has also been used for benign neoplasms, which grow locally, compressing the adjacent tissues, but do not cause distant metastases, that is, they do not spread to other sites of the body. Although benign neoplasms also produce tumor markers, such markers, with a few exceptions, have no clinical significance in the treatment and follow-up of the patient. These markers are physiologically normal substances produced by normal differentiated tissues, and they appear in circulation in excessive amounts.

Physiologically normal substances are produced by malignant neoplasms also, but in addition to the expected gene products there may appear some that are not appropriate for the developmental phase of the organism or the specific kind of tumor tissue.

There are many reports of substances that appear to be unique to malignant neoplasms. However, many claims of tumor-specific gene products, in extended studies, have been proven to be unfounded. This became evident with the application of powerful analytical methods such as radioimmunoassay (RIA) and immunohistochemistry. Small amounts of such substances were found in normal tissues. They more frequently appeared to be phase-specific gene products.

In the literature and in practical use, tumor markers have been called *antigens*. This common usage originated from immunological methods used in the detection and characterization of tumor markers, as well as on the basis of the studies of immunological phenomena associated with such markers. Some of these markers, especially gene products expressed during embryonal development, are in fact weak antigens. They do not elicit in the host any appreciable cellular or humoral immune response. Some of them, with minor variations, are shared by different species.

Tumor markers can be classified in the following three groups: oncofetal, tumor-associated, and tumor-specific (Klavins, 1982a). Each group can be subdivided into universal markers and markers with a limited distribution (Klavins, 1982b).

1

Types of Tumor Markers

ONCOFETAL GENE PRODUCTS

Morphological studies have revealed a striking similarity between embryonic cells and tumor cells. Both cell types have a relatively large nuclear cytoplasmic ratio, they produce a variety of daughter cells, and they are continuously dividing. In the latter aspect, embryonic cells eventually undergo ordinary differentiation to form defined functional organs, whereas tumor cells may differentiate to a certain degree without formation of functional tissues or defined gross anatomical structures.

A special kind of embryonal cells—trophoblasts, which make up the outer layer of the placenta—invades the adjacent tissues, thus mimicking malignant neoplasms. Therefore, the trophoblast may serve as a model to study the biological events of invasiveness. The morphological phenotypic similarity between embryonal cells and tumor cells was observed as early as 1874 by Durante.

More recently, it became evident that there is also a biochemical similarity between embryonal cells and cancer cells of animals and humans. Such well-known phase-specific gene products as α-fetal protein (AFP) (Bergstrand and Czar, 1956) and carcinoembryonic antigen (CEA) (Gold and Freedman, 1965) are produced by a wide variety of malignant neoplasms.

On the basis of such morphological and biochemical observations, the pathogenesis of malignant neoplasms can be considered as arising from normal undifferentiated cells or by dedifferentiation of already fully or partially differentiated normal cells. In both instances, the carcinogenic process can be considered as a faulty differentiation, where malignancy mimics disturbed ontogeny without formation of physiologically and anatomically predictable, defined structures. Thus phase-specific gene products, such as CEA and AFP and those of oncogenes, become markers for malignant neoplasms.

The significance of phase-specific gene products is not known. By their expression and repression during ontogeny, they may be associated with normal differentiation serving different functions (Manes, 1974), none of which is presently defined. It is possible that some fetal gene products are associated with immunological tolerance, both in normal pregnancy and in malignant neoplasms (McCluskey, 1982).

In malignant neoplasms, the expression of embryonal gene products can be considered a phenomenon of either derepression or nonrepression. It depends on the pathogenesis of the malignant neoplasm. If the partially or fully differentiated cells are transformed into tumor cells and this transformation is accompanied by the appearance of embryonal gene products, the pathogenesis of these markers is derepression. In the partially or fully differentiated cells, such gene products are repressed (Fig. 1). On the other hand, if the undifferentiated normal cells are transformed into malignant neoplasms, nonrepression is the pathogenesis of the presence of embryonal gene products (Fig. 2). There are many such undifferentiated cells in tissues—for example, basal cells in different epithelial tissues, histiocytic elements in bone marrow, and lymph nodes. Morphologically these cells, as indicated in Figure 2, have relatively large nuclei and thus resemble embryonal cells. In contrast, the partially or fully differentiated cells (Fig. 1) have a smaller nuclear/cytoplasmic ratio than do embryonal or undifferentiated normal cells. In cancer cells, the nuclei are usually relatively large, as indicated in the diagrams (Figs. 1 and 2).

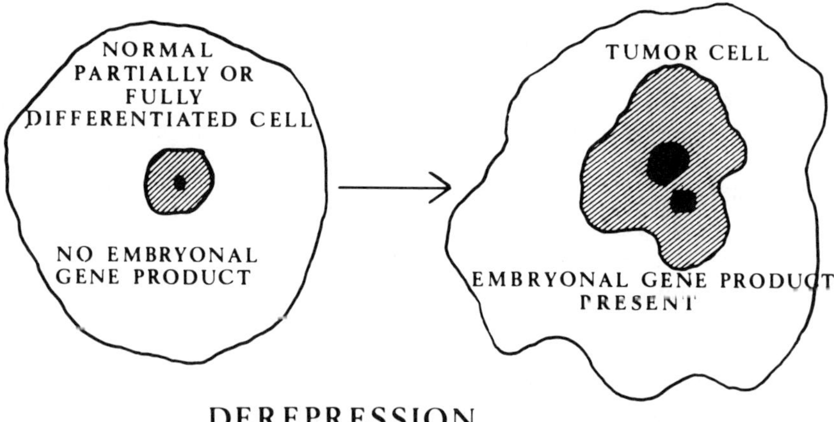

Fig. 1. Transformation of a normal partially or fully differentiated cell into a tumor cell (characterized by irregular shape of cell and nucleus, large nuclear/cytoplasmic ratio, prominent multiple nucleoli). Note the appearance of embryonal gene product, the result of derepression.

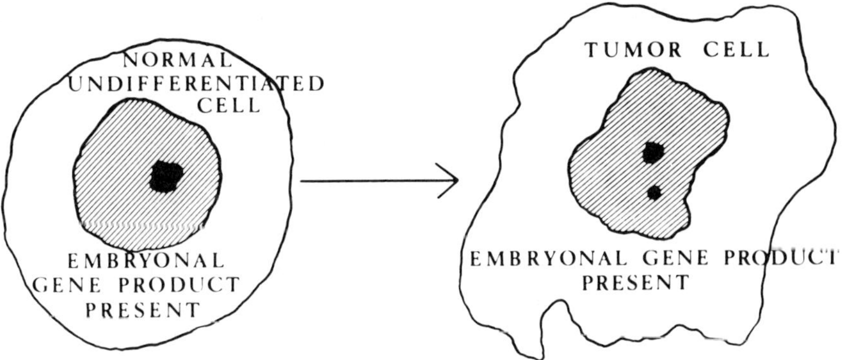

Fig. 2. Transformation of a normal undifferentiated cell (large nuclear/cytoplasmic ratio in comparison with normal partially or fully differentiated cell, Fig. 1.) into a tumor cell (irregular cell and nucleus, multiple nucleoli. Note the appearance of embryonal gene product, the result of nonrepression.

The qualitative and quantitative expressions of various phase-specific gene products are not known. There may be some such entities that appear only briefly during some, probably the earliest, stages of embryogenesis. Subsequently, these gene products may never normally become expressed except in cell transformation. Such gene products could be considered as specific and the most useful tumor markers.

Quantitatively, the usual pattern of the embryonal gene products is such that they decrease with the advance of differentiation, and the adult type of gene products increases, as illustrated in Figure 3. There are two possibilities. One (Fig. 3A) is that certain adult-type gene products are present in the very earliest development, but in small amounts, and increase with time, whereas on the other hand, embryonal gene products decrease as embryogenesis advances. The other possibility, not proven as yet (Fig. 3B), is that certain adult-type gene products are initially absent and certain embryonal antigens later in life are not expressed at all. All the present evidence indicates that small amounts of known embryonal gene products are expressed by undifferentiated normal cells throughout a lifetime. As a consequence of this, the presently known oncofetal gene products are not specific tumor markers even though they are produced in appreciably large amounts by malignant neoplasms.

Oncofetal as well as other gene products used as tumor markers can be divided into two groups, those that are universal and those with a limited distribution (Klavins, 1982b).

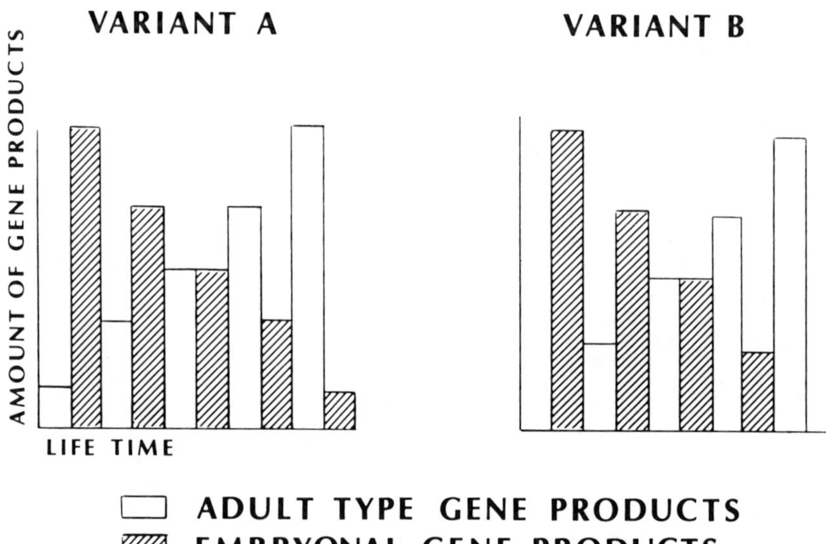

Fig. 3. Production of phase-specific gene products. Variant A: Small amounts of adult-type gene products are expressed at the earliest phases. Subsequently they increase in amount. The embryonal gene products are present in large amounts at the earliest phases; subsequently they decrease. They are present in small amounts even at the latest phases.

Universal Oncofetal Tumor Markers

Universal oncofetal tumor markers are so designated because they appear in embryonic tissues and in malignant neoplasms representing derivatives of all three germinal layers: ectoderm, mesoderm, and entoderm. Some of these gene products have been used clinically and are well defined. The presence of other universal oncofetal gene products is detected by various immunological studies (Klavins et al., 1971), but their nature is not defined. Widely cross-reacting monoclonal antibodies to this type of antigens have been produced by using hybridomas (Seeger et al., 1981). IgM and IgG monoclonal antibodies against midgestational fetal mice tissues cross-reacted with mice, hamsters, and human fetal cells and tumor cells of the same species (Coggin and Payne, 1984).

Carcinoembryonic Antigen (CEA)

CEA is a microheterogeneous glycoprotein. It varies in carbohydrate moiety and in relative proportions of amino acids. Thus, different isolation procedures and sources of CEA may yield various degrees of difference in the measurement of this marker in serum.

Originally CEA was suspected of being a specific gene product occurring only in fetal intestinal mucosa and carcinomas of the intestinal tract (Gold and Freedman, 1965). Now it has been found that tumors other than those derived from entoderm produce CEA—for example, carcinomas of the breast (ectoderm) and uterus (mesoderm). Elevated serum CEA levels are found in patients with chronic bronchitis, chronic pulmonary emphysema, cirrhosis of the liver, regional enteritis, ulcerative colitis, chronic renal disease, cystic fibrosis, and other pancreatic disorders not associated with malignancy. Serum CEA is elevated in heavy smokers of cigarettes, and it increases with age. It is present in normal adult colonic mucosa, but many times less than in carcinoma tissues.

Increased production of CEA or any other oncofetal tumor marker by malignant neoplasms suggests that the neoplastic cells are derived from those few benign counterparts that normally express this gene product. An alternate explanation is that tumor cells produce it as a result of derepression.

Many pathological conditions with increased CEA levels are typical with cell regeneration and hyperplasia, such as cirrhosis of the liver and ulcerative colitis. Thus it is possible that an increased number of normally CEA-producing cells, without alteration in gene expression, may contribute to elevated serum CEA content. Serum of healthy adults contains CEA up to approximately 3 ng/ml.

Because of the wide range of overlap of serum CEA values in different conditions and malignant neoplasms, CEA is not a useful marker for screening purposes. It is valuable in follow-up and during the therapy of patients, especially those with malignant neoplasms of the gastrointestinal tract.

In the interpretation of CEA concentration in sera or tissues it is important to consider cross-reacting substances such as nonspecific cross-reacting antigen 1 (NCA-1) and nonspecific cross-reacting antigen 2 (NCA-2). A biliary glycoprotein I (BGPI) is also known to be related to CEA. With the use of a two-site monoclonal antibody-enzyme immunoassay (MEIA) two epitopes were recognized on the CEA peptide moiety (Hedin et al., 1983). This was accomplished by using two monoclonal antibodies corresponding to these two different epitopes. With this method, no CEA was detected in normal tissue extracts except of the colon. While commercially available CEA assays did not discriminate between CEA and NCA-2, with the MEIA method there was no reaction to this or other CEA-related substances—NCA-1 or BGPI. With this method the CEA concentration in sera of patients with nonmalignant diseases was lower than that obtained with the commercial kits, thus increasing the specificity. The sensitivity was not different from that using the conventional radioimmunoassay of sera from patients with breast, lung, pancreas, and colon carcinomas.

CEA has been used as a model tumor marker to be applied in therapy. Boron-10 labeled antibodies to CEA were found to bind with human colon carcinomas transplanted in hamsters (Goldenberg et al., 1984). This model system provides the ability to study the use of neutron-capture therapy.

α-Fetoprotein (AFP)

This phase-specific gene product was first reported by Bergstrand and Czar (1956) and was subsequently investigated.

AFP is synthesized by yolk sac and liver cells of human fetuses. The size of the corresponding coding genes of AFP and albumin in mice are identical (Kioussis et al., 1981). Therefore, it is suggested that both these genes were derived from a common ancestral gene. Work in our laboratory (Klavins et al., 1974a) and in others indicates that there are several immunologically cross-reacting microheterogeneous species of AFP.

AFP is associated most frequently with hepatomas and yolk sac tumors, both entodermal derivatives. As a universal oncofetal tumor marker, it occurs also in neoplasms derived from ectoderm and mesoderm. For example, elevated serum AFP was found in patients with carcinomas of the uterus (mesodermal derivatives) (Donaldson et al., 1979) and with melanomas (ectodermal derivatives) (Mihalev et al., 1976).

The production of this oncofetal gene product by the malignant neoplasms yolk sac tumor (endodermal sinus tumor) and hepatoma indicates their embryonal character. It is not known which cell types produce AFP in other malignant neoplasms and in some noncancerous conditions, for example, in association with neural tube defects. Adult serum contains 2–20 ng/ml of AFP.

Since AFP is the predominant serum protein in fetuses, most of the functions that are carried out by albumin in adult life can be attributed to AFP during the fetal period. In addition, there is evidence (O'Neill et al., 1981) that AFP may contribute significantly to maintaining self-tolerance during pregnancy.

AFP, like CEA, is a useful tumor marker in monitoring those malignant neoplasms that produce it. Because of the overlap of serum values in patients with malignant neoplasms and in those with noncancerous conditions, it cannot be used for screening purposes. However, AFP in conjunction with a β-subunit of human chorionic gonadotropin can be a significant marker in evaluating the differential diagnosis of germ cell neoplasms (Talerman et al.,

1971). Furthermore, the specificity of the AFP measurements for malignant neoplasms can be increased by use of two high-affinity monoclonal antibodies against separate antigenic sites of AFP (Bellet et al., 1984). By this method serum AFP levels were less than 20 ng/ml in patients with other, noncarcinomatous diseases such as acute and chronic hepatitis and cirrhosis. Serum AFP was greater than 200 ng/ml in 80% of 85 patients with hepatomas.

Tissue Polypeptide Antigen (TPA)

Björklund and Björklund (1957) isolated a species nonspecific antigen (TPA) that was present in different malignant neoplasms and in placenta (Redelius et al., 1980). The main subunit (TPA:β_1) has a molecular weight of 43,000 daltons and contains the antigenic determinant of TPA (Lüning et al., 1980).

It is probably related to cytoskeletal proteins (Kirsch, et al., 1983). The distribution of TPA in normal epithelial tissues (Nathrath and Heidenkummer, 1983) was found to be identical to that of luminal epithelial antigen (Nathrath et al., 1982) associated with intermediate filaments. Although TPA occurs also in sera of healthy individuals, it is significantly higher in patients with malignant neoplasms. It lacks specificity to the same extent as does CEA, but it is useful in monitoring disease processes. TPA as a universal oncofetal tumor marker has been found to have a higher sensitivity than CEA (Klavins and Cho, 1983; Lüthgens and Schlegel, 1983). Furthermore, combined determination of TPA and CEA provided a better discrimination between patients with progressive disease and those with no evidence of disease. The following are the percentage probabilities for a correct discrimination among patients with different malignant neoplasms: colorectal 96%, breast 95%, seminoma 94%, lung 93%, prostate and bladder 90%, renal cell 87%, sarcomas 86%, thyroid 84%, melanomas 83%, head and neck 77%, and female genital tract 76%.

β-Oncofetal Antigen (BOFA)

BOFA was obtained from a colon carcinoma by Sephadex G-200 fractionation of an aqueous extract and subsequent DEAE-cellulose column chromatography (Fritsch and Mach, 1975). Its molecular weight is between 70,000 and 90,000, and it has β-2-mobility and an isoelectric pH between 6 and 7. BOFA is present predominantly in colon carcinoma and in lesser amounts in a wide variety of other malignant neoplasms. It has been detected in different fetal tissues and in smaller quantities—about 10 times less—in normal adult tissues. Immunologically, BOFA was found not to be related to AFP or CEA.

γ-Fetoprotein (GFP)

This universal oncofetal antigen has γ-mobility. Using human serum with breast carcinoma-associated antibodies, Edynak et al. (1972) detected GFP by the Ouchterlony method in a wide variety of human malignant neoplasms as well as in the serum of man, pig, cat, dog, and cow. By the gel immunodiffusion method, this marker was not detected in normal adult tissues or sera of normal subjects and patients with nonmalignant diseases. GFP was present in the jejunum of a patient with intestinal infarcts and in the ileum of a patient with ulcerative colitis, but it was not detected in 99 other tissue samples of different diseased organs. It was demonstrated in the serum in only eight of 1,518 cancer patients.

Basic Fetoprotein (BFP)

This marker has been found in fetal serum and in an extract of fetal intestine (Ishii, 1978). It has a molecular weight of 124,000, γ-electrophoretic mobility; and an isoelectric point of 9.3. Because of its isoelectric point, it has been called basic fetoprotein. BFP was purified from ascites of a patient with hepatoma affinity chromotography, isoelectric focusing, and gel filtration. With a radioimmunoassay technique and a monospecific antibody, it was demonstrated in the sera of normal individuals at a concentration of less than 100 ng/ml. In 180 sera of 240 patients with various nonmalignant diseases, the BFP values were less than 200 ng/ml. In 94 sera of 251 patients with malignant neoplasms, BFP exceeded 200 ng/ml. This marker has a potential usefulness in clinical medicine.

β-S–Fetoprotein

This is a glycoprotein with a molecular weight of approximately 200,000 and β-immunoelectrophoretic mobility. It is heat-resistant to 56°C for 120 min and can be precipitated with ammonium sulfate at 33–50% saturation (Wade et al., 1970).

This marker was obtained from an aqueous extract of a hepatoma, and it is also synthesized by fetal liver (Takahashi et al., 1967). Its universal nature is evident from its presence in the sera of patients with hepatoma, with gastric, colonic, and bronchial carcinomas, with lymphomas, and with leukemias. It has also been found, by the gel immunodiffusion method, in sera during the postpartum period.

Cytoplasmic Antigen (S_2)

This tumor marker was originally thought to be present only in sarcomas. Subsequent studies revealed that S_2 is an oncofetal gene product present in a wide variety of human neoplasms and embryonic tissues (Mukherji and Hirshaut, 1973).

Oncofetal Membrane Antigen (OFA)

OFA was found to be present in a melanoma tissue culture cell line, M14 (Irie et al., 1976). Antisera from patients with malignant melanoma and this cell line as an antigen source were used to study the distribution of OFA by the immune adherence method. It was found in a wide variety of malignant neoplasms and in fetal tissue, notably fetal brain. This antigen was not present in normal adult tissues, except for cultured adult skin and muscle cells.

The distribution and incidence of OFA as determined by the immune adherence absorption technique was found to be as follows: 82% of melanomas, 61% of sarcomas, 53% of breast carcinomas, 71% of lung tumors, 58% of brain tumors, and 11% of colorectal carcinomas were OFA positive (Rees et al., 1981). OFA also induced significant humoral immune response in the host, a property that is not common in other oncofetal markers. It was possible to produce *in vitro* a human IgM antibody to this OFA (Irie et al., 1981).

An antigen known as OFA-I-1 has been found to be expressed by fetal brain and various human malignant neoplasms (Cahan et al., 1982). Another antigen, OFA-I-2, has been found only in tumors of neuroectodermal origin and has been identified as a cell-surface glycolipid-ganglioside, GD2. Chemically it was GalNAcβ1$\rightarrow$4NeuAcα8NeuAcα2$\rightarrow$3Galβ1$\rightarrow$4Glc$\rightarrow$uramide. A monoclonal antibody to OFA-I-2 would appear to be a useful reagent for attempts at immunotherapy (Kawano et al., 1983).

Ganglioside GM2

This universal oncofetal tumor marker is chemically identified as GalNAcβ1$\rightarrow$4NeuAcα2$\rightarrow$3Galβ1$\rightarrow$4GlcCer (Tai et al., 1983). It was detected by nonspecific antibodies produced *in vitro* by B-lymphoblastoid cell lines transformed with Epstein-Barr virus. GM2 is one of the major gangliosides of human fetal brain. Small amounts have been found in fetal liver and adult brain. It has been found in various malignant neoplasms including melanomas, brain tumors, and sarcomas. GM2 is evidently related to or part of the OFA detected in a melanoma tissue culture line, M14 (Irie et al., 1976; Rees et al., 1981).

Interspecies Embryonic Antigen (IEA)

Antisera have been obtained using the protein fraction of amniotic fluid glycoproteins from cattle fetuses (Kalashnikov et al., 1983). Some such antisera were directed to an antigen with a molecular weight of approximately 80,000 daltons, designated as IEA-1. This antigen was detected in the serum of 14–20% of patients with malignant tumors and 58% of those with melanomas. A study using an immunoenzymatic method did not detect IEA in patients free of malignant neoplasms. Another such study did detect an antigen (1EA-2) with a molecular weight of approximately 36,000 daltons in sera of 21–22% of cancer patients as well as in patients free of malignant tumors.

Stage-Specific Embryonic Antigen (SSEA-1)

This is another interspecies phase-specific embryonic antigen. SSEA-1 is a gene product of murine preimplantation embryos and is expressed by human embryonal carcinoma cells. Human blood group antigen I is related to it and is produced by mice embryos also. Human granulocytes contain SSEA-1, while I is present on human erythrocytes according to Knowles et al. (1982). SSEA-1 was found in different malignant neoplasms as well as in normal human and mouse tissues by Fox et al (1983). SSEA-1 was also expressed in breast and ovarian carcinomas. Normal breast and ovarian tissues were SSEA-1-negative.

DNA-Binding Proteins

Two species of human serum DNA-binding protein make up this group of oncofetal tumor markers (Parsons et al., 1978).

Serum DNA-binding protein (BIP)

This unique protein inhibits the degradation of DNA by bleomycin and has a molecular weight of 64,000 daltons and a pI of 5.9 (Galvan et al., 1982). Assays for bleomycin inhibitor protein have revealed it to be markedly decreased in serum of patients with various solid tumors, leukemias, and lymphomas.

C3DP

This is a human serum DNA-binding glycoprotein and a fragment of the complement component C3. It was isolated from fetal cord serum by Parsons and Hoch (1976). C3DP has a molecular weight of 135,000 and consists of three subunits, 74,000, 40,000, and 22,000 daltons. It is present in an appreciable amount in fetal cord serum and sera from patients with malignant neoplasms, representing all three germinal derivatives (Parsons and Kowal, 1978). While the sera of normal individuals contain up to approximately 150 μg/ml of C3DP, in the sera of patients with malignant neoplasms these values range from 150 to 400 μg/ml. Measurements of serum C3DP have been valuable indicators for monitoring the disease processes.

MAD-2

This is another DNA-binding protein that is an oncofetal tumor marker. It was isolated from human serum (Parsons et al., 1979) and consists of a 200,000–210,000 molecular weight single polypeptide chain. MAD-2 is immunologically different from C3DP. It is immunologically identical with plasma fibronectin and may represent a fragment of it. This marker has the same potential significance as C3DP. It has been demonstrated in sera of patients with a wide variety of malignant neoplasms and also in sera of fetal cord, pregnant women, and, in a lesser concentration, some healthy individuals (Parsons and Kowal, 1978).

The Serum Globulin T-Globulin

T-globulin has been found in sera of pregnant women and cancer patients with various malignant neoplasms including sarcomas, lymphomas, and leukemias (Tal and Halperin, 1970). With the immunoelectrophoresis method it was not detected in the sera of patients with nonneoplastic conditions. Apparently, there is a tumor cell surface factor ceramide-lactoside (cytolipin H) that specifically binds T-globulin.

Isoenzymes

Many isoenzymes are phase-specific gene products occurring during a certain period of development or produced by certain embryonic tissues. Embryonic isoenzymes reappear in malignant neoplasms (Criss, 1971). The enzyme pattern of fast-growing tumors resembles more closely the pattern of the embryonic period than does that of slowly growing, well-differentiated neoplasms.

Regan isoenzyme

An alkaline phosphatase, Regan isoenzyme has been well investigated (Fishman et al., 1971). It is a heat-stable glycoprotein present in placenta and in cell membranes of different human malignant neoplasms. This tumor marker appears in increased amounts in sera of patients with breast, bronchial, intestinal, and biliary carcinomas and with lymphomas.

Elevated serum levels are associated with tissue regeneration, and some healthy individuals also have elevated values. There are several variants of this isoenzyme. It has antigenic determinants in common with intestinal alkaline phosphatase (Lehmann, 1975). One isoenzyme—testicular placenta-like alkaline phosphatase—may be a variant of Regan isoenzyme that is expressed in malignant neoplasms (Millan and Stigbrand, 1983). In addition, there are other species of alkaline phosphatase related to fetal or tumor tissue gene products (Fishman, 1980). For example, L-homoarginine-sensitive alkaline phosphatase is an early placental isoenzyme, Nago isoenzyme is present in term placenta and carcinomas of ovary and lung, and Kasahara isoenzyme is present in hepatomas and fetal intestine.

There are several possible variations of the placental form of alkaline phosphatase (Loose et al., 1984). The reaction of monoclonal antibodies to placental alkaline phosphatase has been found to be restricted to fewer malignant neoplasms than the reaction of polyclonal antibodies. There may be alteration in the gene, the transcription, or the translation product, or cross-reactivity with some other entity.

Isoferritins

In fetal liver there have been found isoferritins similar to those of placenta, a hepatoma, and HeLa cells (Drysdale and Alpert, 1975). They have a more acidic isoelectric point than ferritins from normal adult tissues (McFarlane et al., 1980). Such unique isoferritins have been detected in sera of patients with other malignant neoplasms as well as in some normal individuals (Mori et al., 1975).

Fetal thymidine kinase

This fetal isoenzyme is different from the adult-type enzyme and appears in human malignant neoplasms (Stafford and Jones, 1972).

Fetal Liver Ferroprotein **(**α_2-HF)

This marker is synthesized by fetal liver. Its serum concentration decreases after birth but reappears in patients with a wide variety of malignant neoplasms: gastric, intestinal, pulmonary, mammary, and hepatic carcinomas, and Ewing sarcomas and lymphomas. Elevated serum levels can occur also in patients with nonneoplastic diseases. Like AFP, it is produced predominantly by hepatomas, but it can be present in increased amounts in sera of patients with other liver diseases, such as cirrhosis.

This oncofetal marker is a glycoferroprotein with a molecular weight of 600,000. Buffe and Rimbaut (1975) observed that α_2-HF cross-reacted immunologically with ferritin but was not identical to it. α_2–HF inhibited mitogen- and antigen-induced lymphoblastic transformation.

Pregnancy-Associated α_2-Glycoprotein (α_2-PAG)

Due to variability of this marker in the serum of pregnant women, healthy individuals, and patients with malignant neoplasms, the value of serial α_2-PAG determinations is solely in the follow-up studies (Bauer, 1981).

Human Fetal Antigen (HFA)

An aqueous extract of a 6- to 7-week-old intact human fetus was used as the antigen to raise an immune serum in a rabbit (Klavins et al., 1971). After appropriate absorption with normal tissues this antiserum cross-reacted with human malignant neoplasms, representing derivatives of all three germinal layers. Using fluorescence microscopy, Mesa-Tejada et al. (1972a) demonstrated that the localization of this antigen in colon carcinoma was similar to that of CEA. In other carcinomas, too, the localization was predominantly in the periphery of tumor cells.

This human fetal antigen, after fractionation on a Sephadex G-200, yielded a component with a molecular weight of approximately 60,000 (Klavins et al., 1974a). Antiserum to this fraction (HFA_1) had a more limited cross-reactivity with different tumor extracts than did the antiserum to the crude extract (HFA). Following further purification of HFA_1 with CM-Cellex ion exchange chromatography, a homogeneous component was obtained as noted on polyacrylamide gel electrophoresis. However, it appeared microheterogeneous on isoelectric focusing within a pH range of 4.2–5.2, and antiserum to it cross-reacted only with extracts of a hepatoma and a carcinoma of the pancreas.

With a different approach, human fetal extracts were tested by macrophage electrophoretic mobility (MEMB) against white blood cells from cancer patients and controls (Pasternak et al., 1982). A positive MEMB reaction was obtained in 73% of 284 patients with various malignant neoplasms. Among 134 controls, the positive rate was 11%. There was a cross-reaction between human and mouse fetal extracts. Lymphocytes from pregnant women also reacted with fetal extracts.

Leukocyte migration was inhibited in 75% of 65 tumor patients and 14% of 50 controls, and leukocyte adherence was inhibited in 80% of 50 cancer patients and in 19% of 54 controls.

It appears from these studies that there are common fetal and tumor-associated substances.

Human Placental Antigen

Placenta is easily obtained and may substitute for other embryonic tissues in the study of oncofetal tumor markers. A rabbit immune serum was raised with a placenta from a 3.5-cm human fetus. By means of Ouchterlony double-diffusion technique, it was seen that this antiserum, appropriately absorbed with normal adult tissues, cross-reacted with extracts of an adenocarcinoma of the pancreas, two well-differentiated adenocarcinomas of the colon, and a poorly differentiated squamous cell carcinoma of the esophagus (Mesa-Tejada et al., 1972b). This placental antiserum had more limited cross-reactivity with malignant neoplasms than did the antiserum to whole human embryo (HFA).

This placental antigen was fractionated by Sephadex G-200 gel filtration, and two distinct immunologically active fractions were obtained (Klavins et al., 1974b). One fraction had alkaline phosphatase activity, presumably Regan isoenzyme (Fishman et al., 1971). These two immunologically active fractions were pooled and after cellulose acetate electrophoresis again exhibited two major fractions.

Tn Antigen

This antigen is the precursor in the biosynthesis of a tumor-associated antigen T (Springer, 1984). Tn and T are precursors of blood group MN antigens. Both these antigens are masked in normal cells but become unmasked in tumor cells and serve as universal markers. Tn has been demonstrated immunohistochemically in a wide variety of malignant neoplasms. Both Tn and T occur in early fetal life.

Common Nucleolar Antigen

This antigen is present predominantly in different malignant neoplasms. On isoelectric focusing, it had one major band of a pI of 6.3 and a minor one at a pI of 6.1 (Busch et al., 1981). A high degree of accuracy was obtained in the differentiation of malignant and benign breast lesions by immunofluorescence microscopy with an antiserum to nucleolar extracts. Since purified antibodies to tumor nucleolar antigens reacted weakly with extracts from human placenta (Kelsey et al., 1981) and a fetal fibroblast cell line (P.K. Chan et al., 1983), they are oncofetal antigens.

Oncofetal Markers With a Limited Distribution

Tumor markers of this group do not occur in malignant neoplasms representing derivatives of all three germinal layers but are produced predominantly by one kind of tissue. These markers will be considered along with tumor-associated and putative tumor-specific ones in sections dealing with malignant neoplasms of specific tissues or organ systems.

TUMOR-ASSOCIATED MARKERS

These gene products are substances produced by differentiated or partially differentiated cells of an adult organism. They occur in increased amounts in association with malignant neoplasms either as an increased synthesis by the tumor cells or as an increased plasma concentration because of an increased number of tumor cells producing such substances. Like oncofetal markers, these tumor markers can be divided into two groups—universal tumor-associated markers and those with a limited distribution.

Universal Tumor-Associated Markers

Any one of these tumor markers, mostly well-known gene products, may occur in patients with different malignant neoplasms, representing derivatives of all three germinal layers. They are produced by nonmalignant or normal adult tissues also, but at lower serum concentrations and less frequently than in sera of patients with malignant neoplasms.

Hormones as Tumor-Associated Markers

Ectopic production of hormones is a general phenomenon of genetic derepression of hormone transcripts or differentiation of tumors in a certain direction with production of hormones. A variety of hormones are associated with malignant neoplasms (Pimentel, 1983). Some of them arise within a limited group of tumors, others are produced by single, distinct malignant neoplasms. Besides increased production, qualitative changes can occur in these tumor-produced hormones (Pimentel, 1983). Prostaglandins are a group of hormones elevated in the serum of patients with different malignant neoplasms (B.J. Smith, et al., 1983).

Many malignant neoplasms express ACTH and other pituitary hormones. By the use of antisera to hormones as tumor markers pituitary adenomas have been classified in two groups: adenomas with hormone secretion and adenomas without secretory activity (Garancis et al., 1983). This approach provides more specific information about any tumor with expression of a specific product.

CA19-9

This is a colon carcinoma cell surface antigen. A comparison was made between CEA and CA19-9 as to the sensitivity and specificity in marking different malignant neoplasms (Gupta et al., 1983). CA19-9 was more sensitive for pancreatic and bile duct carcinomas and CEA for colon, breast, and gastric carcinomas. Assuming a normal serum concentration of 30 ng/ml, elevated serum levels were measured in 79% of 80 patients with pancreatic,

46% of 24 with gastric, 46% of 164 with advanced colorectal, and 8% with local carcinomas (Del Villano et al., 1983). With this normal value false elevation of serum CA19-9 levels was observed in 0.6% of 1,020 blood donors.

The Glycoprotein JBB5

This marker was isolated from the urine of a patient with carcinoma of the colon (Chawla et al., 1977). It migrated as an α_1-globulin and had a molecular weight between 51,000 and 59,000. By the double-immunodiffusion method JBB5 was found predominantly in the urine of patients with metastatic colonic carcinomas and less frequently in the urine of patients with other malignant neoplasms. It was present in 4% of sera from patients with various nonmalignant diseases. This marker was not tested for cross-reactivity with fetal tissues.

α_1-Acid Glycoprotein (AGP)

Serum AGP was found by radioimmunoassay to be elevated in 89% of 190 patients with solid tumors and 87% of 58 with hematologic neoplasms (Ganz et al., 1983). Among 71 patients with diseases other than malignant neoplasms, there were 18% with elevated serum AGP. Especially in patients with lung, pancreas, and colon carcinomas, and with lymphomas, serum AGP determinations could serve to monitor the effects of therapy and the course of the disease.

Basic Polypeptide (F_2A_1)

This polypeptide was isolated from a histone of a calf thymus. When it was used in a macrophage electrophoretic mobility test (Fish, 1973), it was possible to discriminate between lymphocytes of cancer patients and those of normal individuals. A component of F_2A_1 was absent or was associated with lymphocytes of healthy people in significantly lesser amounts. Tests for the presence of F_2A_1 in fetal cells have not been reported.

Serum Sialic Acid

Elevated serum protein and sialic acid levels have been associated with the presence of malignant neoplasms. Determination of these parameters in serum was found to be useful in the monitoring of cancer patients during treatment (Harvey et al., 1981). When there was a good response to therapy they decreased, and in recurrence they became elevated. Serum sialic acid was elevated in cancer patients with a mean concentration of 2.99 μM/ml, whereas in normal control serum it was 1.74 μM/ml (Shamberger, 1983).

Elevated serum levels have been observed also in psoriasis, Crohns disease, and some inflammatory diseases. However, in comparison with CEA sialic acid has appeared to be more sensitive as a tumor marker. It indicates the effectiveness of therapy by decreasing to normal levels.

Lipid-associated sialic acid (LSA) has been considered a universal tumor-associated marker with a normal serum level up to 20 mg% (Katopodis et al., 1983). In cancer patients, the serum levels exceeded 20 mg% in 86% to 100% of cases depending on the kind of tumor. The sensitivity increased from 1% to 12% if the serum samples were not stored but analyzed immediately. As is the case with CEA, smoking also affected the serum levels of LSA. The mean value for smokers was 19.4 mg% (Hirshaut et al., 1983). Lipid-associated sialic acid was a better indicator of malignancy than the total serum sialic acid (Horgan, 1982). In combined use LSA and CEA supplemented each other as universal tumor markers (Munjal et al., 1983). The highest levels of serum LSA occurred in patients with lung cancer, followed by colorectal and other tumors, the lowest occurring in breast cancer patients. CEA was highest, as expected, in colon carcinoma patients, followed by other tumors, lung, and breast.

Lactosylsphingosine

Antibodies to lactosylsphingosine occur at a significantly higher level in cancer patients than in normal individuals (Jozwiak and Koscielak, 1980). Similarly, elevated antibody levels were found to be present in patients with hemolytic anemia and severe burns. It was suggested that antibodies were produced to lactosylsphingosine present on tumor cell plasma membranes.

The Glycoprotein EDC1

This marker was isolated from the urine of a patient with acute myelogenous leukemia (Rudman et al., 1976). EDC1 has been partially characterized. It occurs in sera of patients with malignant neoplasms at a higher concentration than in patients with nonmalignant diseases, when measured by radioimmunoassay. It is not known if EDC1 occurs in embryonal tissues.

Ca Antigen

A monoclonal antibody (Ca-1) against a hybrid, produced by fusing diploid fibroblasts with cervical carcinoma cells, reacted with an antigen in cell membranes of different human malignant neoplasm cell lines (Ashall et al., 1982). Ca-1 did not react with human diploid cells; however, the antigen was present in very low concentration in homogenates of normal adult and fetal tissues. The antigen consisted of two glycoproteins with molecular weights of 350,000 and 390,000. The antigen was designated Ca antigen. Immunohistochemical studies revealed that except for epithelium of oviducts and transitional epithelium of urinary tract, this Ca-1 antibody did not react with other nonneoplastic tissues. Various malignant neoplasms, with the exception of malignant brain tumors, neuroblastomas, melanomas, some lymphomas, some sarcomas, seminomas, testicular teratocarcinomas, and prostatic carcinomas, reacted with the Ca-1. The antigen also occurred, infrequently, in colon and other gastrointestinal carcinomas (McGee et al., 1982). Malignant cells in effusions could be identified by using Ca-1 antibody.

Plasminogen Activator

Malignant neoplasms produce plasminogen activator in significantly increased amounts. It is elevated by a factor of 3–50 in all malignant tissues, compared with corresponding normal tissues (Ossowski and Vassalli, 1978). However, it may be decreased in the plasma. It has been suggested (Colombi et al., 1984) that plasminogen activator in tumor-tissue periphery may promote the invasion.

Fibrinopeptide A (FPA)

In 60% of 43 patients with advanced carcinomas there was evidence of increased blood coagulation (Rickles et al., 1983). FPA in the serum of these patients tended to increase and paralleled the progression of the tumor. Patients with persistently elevated serum FPA values had a poor prognosis.

Lipotropin (LPH)

Serum levels of lipotropin have been found to be elevated in patients with malignant neoplasms (Odell et al., 1979), indicating an ectopic production of LPH by tumor cells. In cancer tissues, LPH was found in higher concentration than in corresponding normal tissues. Among 107 patients with abnormal chest roentgenograms, 36% of 74 patients with subsequently diagnosed lung carcinoma had elevated plasma LPH levels. LPH was also produced by some colon, stomach, breast, renal, prostatic, cervical, and ovarian carcinomas.

Serum Ribonuclease (S-RNase)

This enzyme was compared with CEA as a ptoential screening test for malignant neoplasms (Renner et al., 1979). Serum CEA was elevated in 28% and S-RNase in 85% of patients with various malignant neoplasms (14 breast, 15 lung, 18 colon, 8 hepatomas, and 24 other tumors).

Tumor-Associated Antigen (TAG)

This marker, also known as Tennessee antigen, is a glycoprotein with a molecular weight of 50,000–60,000 (Ramsey et al., 1982). TAG was extracted from an adenocarcinoma of the colon. It is different from CEA and was present in carcinomas of colon, stomach, breast, and ovaries with predominant localization in the plasma membrane area. For gastric carcinomas it had a sensitivity of 71% and a specificity of 77% (Sampson et al., 1982).

Sarcoma-Associated Antigens

Sarcoma-associated antigens have been detected by a complement fixation method and found to be present also in a wide variety of other malignant neoplasms. One of these antigens, S_3, apparently is a heterophile substance and was found in family members of sarcoma patients (Sethi and Hirshaut, 1981).

Creatine Kinase BB (CK-BB)

This isoenzyme may occur in increased amounts in serum of patients with various malignant neoplasms (Rubery et al., 1982). Among 1,015 patients with malignant neoplasms it was elevated in 41% of bronchogenic carcinomas and 34% of lymphomas (Rubery et al., 1982). Serum CK-BB was elevated and correlated with the clinical course of patients with breast, ovarian, uterus, cervix, stomach, and intestinal carcinomas, as well as with sarcomas. In patients with prostatic, testicular, bladder, and head and neck carcinomas, serum CK-BB was elevated more frequently in association with metastic disease than with any local involvement.

Neuron-Specific Enolase (NSE)

NSE is a glycolytic enzyme. It consists of α, β, and γ subunits, the γ subunit being the so-called nervous-system-specific protein. The γ subunit is species-nonspecific. The enolase in brain consists of 3 isoenzymes composed of $\alpha\,\alpha$, $\alpha\,\gamma$, and $\gamma\,\gamma$, the last two constituting the NSE. This NSE is produced by normal neuroendocrine cells and neuroendocrine tumors. Thus it serves as a tumor marker that differentiates the histologic types, and if elevated in serum it can be used as a marker for follow-up of the platients. NSE is produced by neuroblastomas, carcinoids, insulinomas, glucagonomas, medullary carcinomas of thyroid, some adenocarcinomas of colon, and small-cell carcinomas of lung. Production of NSE by small-cell carcinomas of lung, for example, sets this tumor apart from other lung carcinomas (Ariyoshi et al., 1983b).

Galactosyltransferase

This enzyme was found elevated in the serum of patients with breast, ovarian, respiratory tract, and gastrointestinal tract carcinomas (Capel et al.,

1982). The most marked enzyme concentration was noted in association with breast carcinomas. Serum isoenzyme II concentration was especially related to different malignant neoplasms (Pohl et al., 1983).

Galactosyltransferase isoenzymes

At least 1 of 5 isoenzymes was found to be elevated in serum of 79% of patients with different malignant neoplasms by Davey et al., 1984. On the other hand, an isoenzyme with a pI of 5.1 was not found in the sera of patients with a hepatoma (Qian et al., 1984).

Sialyltransferase (ST)

ST levels have been found to be above normal in sera of patients with solid tumors such as breast, colon, and lung carcinomas, melanomas, and tumors of the lymphoreticular system. The concentration was related to tumor burden, and the enzyme determinations provided considerable information about the clinical course of the disease (Pohl et al., 1983).

Serum Fucose (F) and Fucosyl Transferase Activity (FT)

Both F and FT are universal tumor-associated markers. They occurred at a high concentration in serum of patients, studied by Sen et al. (1983), with a wide range of malignant neoplasms. With a few exceptions F and FT levels were parallel.

Gangliosides

Two major gangliosides, characterized as A and B, were detected in a human hepatoma and a colon carcinoma and isolated by using a monoclonal antibody to sailosyl alpha 2 leads to 6 galactosyl residue (Hakomori et al., 1983). A third ganglioside had a ceramide nonasaccharide structure. After desialylation it reacted to anti-X-hapten antibody. These three gangliosides have been found in some normal tissues in considerably smaller quantities than in malignant neoplasms.

Unconjugated Pteridins

There is a significantly higher excretion of urinary xanthopterin, neopterin, and pterin in cancer patients than in healthy adults, according to Stea et al. (1981), who found that these markers could be used to monitor the clinical course of cancer patients. The pteridine concentration in urine corresponded to the stage of the disease in patients with Hodgkin's lymphoma. Among patients with different malignant neoplasms urinary pteridine measurements were helpful in the evaluation of those with tumors of the female genital tract.

Polyamines

The polyamines putresine, spermine, and spermidine are excreted in the urine of cancer patients in higher amounts than in that of control groups (Sadananda et al., 1980). Such an increase was observed in 75% of 81 patients studied. Rapid estimation of plasma polyamines was possible using gas chromatography (Bakowski et al., 1981). It was useful in clinical studies, especially in the follow-up of cancer patients. Polyamines have not, however, proved to be useful markers for colon carcinomas (Carachi and Beeley, 1983). Urinary excretion was not statistically significantly different from that of controls. On the other hand, polyamine levels in urine have been useful in monitoring the disease state of patients with breast, stomach, prostate, female genital tract, and metastatic carcinomas of unknown origin (Horn et al., 1982).

Modified Nucleosides

Urinary excretion of modified nucleosides, especially pseudouridine (ψrd) is correlated with the course of malignant neoplastic diseases (Salvatore et al., 1983a). The modified nucleosides are derived from tRNA by several processes, e.g. increased turnover of some species or alterations of tRNA-modifying enzymes in malignant neoplasms (Borek et al., 1983).

A test for serum concentration of pseudouridine was developed to avoid the influence of external variables (Salvatore et al., 1983b). It was found that serum ψrd concentrations varied between 1.64 and 12.05 nμ/ml in patients with a wide variety of malignant neoplasms including leukemias and lymphomas. These values exceeded the normal mean value by at least two standard deviations.

C1 Esterase Inhibitor

This complement 1 esterase inhibitor protein was found by Abad and Lluch, Jr., (1980) to be elevated in the serum of cancer patients and correlated with the clinical stage of the disease.

β_2-Microglobulin

This protein is associated with many different malignant neoplasms—breast carcinomas (Weiss et al., 1981), colon carcinomas, hepatomas, and melanomas (Thomas et al., 1978). When Burkitt lymphoma cells (Ramos) were grown in the presence of human leukocyte interferon (HuIFN-α), there was an increase of β_2-microglobulin on the surface of the cells and in the culture medium (Fellous et al., 1981). This indicates increased synthesis of β_2-microglobulin by the cells.

Ferritin

There is evidence that tumor cells may synthesize increased amounts of ferritin. Thus it was possible to detect leukemia involvement by finding elevated ferritin levels in cerebrospinal fluid (Dillmann et al., 1982). Furthermore, it is possible that tumor cells produce ferritin that differs from that of normal-tissue ferritin. Hybridoma antibodies produced to pancreatic carcinoma ferritin do not react with normal liver ferritin (Ruppert et al., 1984). There is an increase in the number of ferritin-bearing lymphocytes in the peripheral blood of cancer patients, as demonstrated by Papenhausen et al. (1984). In their study the mean percentage of such lymphocytes was 10% in cancer patients and 3.1% in the controls.

Epidermal Growth Factor (EGF)

Some malignant neoplasms such as lung and pancreatic carcinomas, produce EGF, as shown by Okano et al. (1982). In various normal tissues examined, Brunner's glands of duodenum and acini of submandibular glands contained EGF. It is possible that EGF can be a marker for some malignant neoplasms.

Cytokeratins

With cytokeratins—a group of intermediate filaments—as tumor-associated markers, it is possible to differentiate into subgroups morphologically similar-looking carcinomas (Debus et al., 1984). It is not known whether such differentiation is significant clinically. In several instances these markers, e.g. human cytokeratin No. 18, may facilitate differential diagnosis. A monoclonal antibody bank has been developed (Debus et al., 1984) for each intermediate filament type.

Transforming Growth Factor (TGF)

The activity of TGF is associated with the expression of malignant phenotypes. High-molecular-weight TGF (M_r 30,000–35,000), which coelutes with epidermal growth factor competing activity, was present in urine in 82% of 22 cancer patients and 23% of controls examined by Sherwin et al. (1983). This TGF activity in urine may be considered a universal tumor marker.

S-100 Proteins

These proteins, depending on which of two subunits is involved, are predominantly present in glial cells but also occur in melanocytes, adipocytes, chondrocytes, and other nonneural cells. Recently S-100a protein consisting of two α subunits was detected in blood monocytes, macrophages of lymph nodes, alveolar macrophages, and Kupffer cells (Takahashi et al., 1984). S-100b protein was present in Langerhans cells, interdigitating reticulum cells, and histiocytosis X cells.

Tumor-Associated Markers With a Limited Distribution

These markers are limited to a single or few malignant neoplasms and the corresponding normal adult tissues. They will be discussed in the chapters concerned with malignant neoplasms of specific tissues or organ systems, along with oncofetal and putative tumor-specific markers.

TUMOR-SPECIFIC MARKERS

Tumor-specific markers would have to be unique gene products representing altered genomes; the biological behavior of malignant neoplasms suggests that genetic alterations have indeed occurred in the normal cells.

The sites and extent of these alterations are, with the exception of a few oncogenes, not presently known. There are no well-established tumor-specific markers that can be used in clinical medicine, in spite of many reports about such gene products in man and animals. Some of the suggested specific markers may turn out on further study to be either oncofetal or tumor-associated gene products.

These markers can also be divided into two groups, universal tumor-specific markers and those with a limited distribution.

Universal Tumor-Specific Markers

Expression of a gene product that is identical in different malignant neoplasms derived from all three germinal layers would indicate that carcinogenesis is associated with a unique genetic alteration. Such substances have been suggested. Patients with different malignant neoplasms were studied in regard to leukocyte migration inhibition (LMI) by neoplastic antigens (Mantovani et al., 1981). It was concluded that the LMI response of cancer patients is not tissue-specific, nor is it directed to a specific tumor-associated antigen but rather to a wide range of antigens shared by several types of tumors.

Malignolipin

One of the earliest identified tumor markers, malignolipin, has been suggested as a specific component of malignant neoplasms (Kosaki et al., 1958). It is a spermine-containing phospholipid.

A Urinary Protein

Aron et al. (1974) reported that there is a tumor-specific protein in the urine of cancer patients. The protein was found in urine of patients with a wide variety of malignant neoplasms but not in the urine of individuals without malignant disease.

A Common Tumor Antigen (CTA)

Basic membrane protein is a peptide that has appeared as a common tumor antigen (CTA) in plasma membranes of tumor cells (Dickinson et al., 1976). This marker was related to a normal tissue antigen (NTA) and "the basic protein of myelin." It has a molecular weight of about 17,000. CTA can be extracted from the cell membranes with proteolipid solvents and acid below a pH of 3.0. This marker was found in a wide variety of malignant neoplasms including leukemias and sarcomas.

Proteolytic Procoagulant (CPA)

Malignant neoplasms contain a unique proteolytic procoagulant (CPA), which was found to differ from tissue thromboplastin in that it was not dependent on factor VII but initiated coagulation directly by factor X activation (Gordon, 1981). CPA was inhibited by diisopropylfluorophosphate, whereas tissue thromboplastin was not. It is a cysteine protease with a molecular weight of 68,000 daltons and isoelectric point of 4.8–4.9. In general, procoagulant activity was found to be abundantly present in plasma membrane vesicles shed from tumor cells (Dvorak et al., 1982).

B-Protein

This marker protein, present in the sera of cancer patients, has been so designated because it interacts with a low-molecular-weight binding protein of Baker's yeast (Bucovaz et al., 1978). The assay of B-protein is based on this property. B-protein of patients is similar to B-protein produced by the spleen of New Zealand white rabbits. Serum B-protein levels have reflected the course of the disease. There is a normal serum protein counterpart, which can be converted *in vitro* to a protein with properties similar to those of the B-protein (Macleod et al., 1984).

Malignancy-Associated Glycoprotein

A unique glycoprotein with a molecular weight of approximately 50,000–55,000 was isolated from pooled plasma of cancer patients (Delong Bolmer and Davidson, 1981). From the preliminary investigations, it appears that this glycoprotein was not a normal serum component nor was it related to any of the known tumor antigens.

Tumor Amylases

Amylase isoenzymes were isolated by Takeuchi et al., (1981) from a bronchoalveolar carcinoma, an epithelial thymoma, and a serous papillary cystadenocarcinoma of the ovary. Although immunologically identical with pancreatic and salivary amylases, the tumor amylases had a different amino acid composition.

Tumor-Specific tRNAs

These tRNAs are formed by modified nucleosides. In tumor tRNA the species hydroxy Y base is hypomodified by lacking methyl and carboxymethyl groups (Nishimura et al., 1982). This base analog could be a useful tumor marker. Quenosine at the first position of the anticodon was found to have been replaced by guanosine in all tumor cells tested. Q-base analogs can be synthesized and incorporated into the tumor cell tRNA for diagnostic and therapeutic purposes.

Antigens Detected by Monoclonal Antibodies

Monoclonal antibodies against an osteogenic sarcoma produced by hybridomas, in a study by Embleton et al. (1981), reacted not only with other osteogenic sarcoma cells but also with cell lines derived from carcinomas of the colon, lung, bladder, and cervix. They did not cross-react with normal cells. Similarly, hybridoma monoclonal antibodies produced to a human lung carcinoma cell line cross-reacted with a wide variety of malignant neoplasms (Kasai et al., 1981). A monoclonal antibody to a lung tumor line immunoprecipitated a common antigen from different malignant neoplasms but not from normal fibroblasts (Pak et al., 1983).

Tumor-Specific Markers With a Limited Distribution

There is evidence from animal experiments that malignant neoplasms produce some unique tumor-specific gene products. Cloned C3H mouse embryonic cells after transformation with chemical carcinogens produced unique antigens for each of eight transformed lines (Embleton and Heidelberger, 1975). Some studies of human malignant neoplasms have been interpreted to indicate that there is no common specific antigen for all human cancers (Korosteleva, 1957).

There are specific antigens shared by tumors of similar histologic type, as determined by cytotoxicity of lymphocytes incubated with immune RNA (Pilch et al., 1976) or by using a modified leukocyte adherence inhibition technique (Rutherford et al. 1977; Thomson et al. 1978).

By using hybridoma-secreted monoclonal antibodies Steplewski and Koprowski (1981) demonstrated unique antigens, located on colorectal carcinoma cells or melanoma cells, as well as antigens shared among melanoma and astrocytoma cells. These markers will be discussed along with oncofetal and tumor-associated markers in chapters dealing with malignant neoplasms of specific tissues or organ systems. It has been questioned whether various monoclonal antibodies thus far produced correspond to true tumor-specific antigens (Thompson et al., 1983a). They are highly selective regarding antigen specificity, but these antigens may be phase-specific normal gene products, normal adult-type products not examined, or products expressed in quantities too small to be detected with available methods.

Various virus-associated markers and the viruses themselves have been considered as tumor markers. If the pathogenesis of malignant neoplasms were to resemble that of infectious disease, the viruses could be considered, similarly to other microorganisms, as specific markers for at least some of the malignant neoplasms. So far there is only one example of a human oncogenic virus—HTLV (Gallo and Wong-Staal, 1982). There are numerous reports of serological cross-reactivity between cancer patients and viruses. Such reactions have to be evaluated carefully before conclusions are made about relationships between malignant neoplasms and viruses. Healthy subjects were shown to contain antibodies to glycoprotein (gp70) of simian sarcoma virus-simian sarcoma-associated virus (Snyder and Fleissner, 1980). These findings were interpreted as the development of antibodies to natural substances with cross-reacting antigens and not as an immunological response to infection by this virus.

2

Carcinomas of Various Organs and Organ Systems

BREAST CANCER

Oncofetal Markers

CEA

By conventional methods CEA was demonstrated by Henderson et al. (1976) at levels above normal in the sera of 42% of patients with breast carcinoma. Of 23 patients who developed breast carcinoma between two mammography screening periods, 65% had histochemically demonstrable CEA (Halter et al., 1982).

High cytosol concentration of CEA was associated with estrogen and progesterone receptor-positive tumors (Goodyear et al., 1983), but plasma CEA did not necessarily correlate with the cytosol values. Therefore low-CEA cytosols with negative steroid receptors and high plasma CEA concentrations might indicate a larger tumor burden than would steroid receptor-positive, high-CEA-containing tumors and low plasma CEA. There was a better response to medical therapy by patients with elevated serum CEA (Palazzo et al., 1984). Only 6.6% of CEA-negative patients responded, compared to 55% of patients with elevated serum CEA.

Elevated serum CEA had a frequency of 8% among 107 patients with recurrence of carcinoma in the chest wall only (Lee, 1983). When metastases occurred in visceral organs or bones, instances of elevated serum CEA levels and the degree of elevation increased considerably.

In a study of 628 patients before and 577 patients after treatment for breast cancer, serum CEA determination was of marginal value in diagnosis or prognosis (Wang et al., 1984).

Similarly, in another study (Mughal et al., 1983) response rates and remissions were not dependent on pretreatment plasma CEA concentration. However, in 94% of patients who responded to chemotherapy plasma CEA decreased. The remission lasted 22 months for those patients whose CEA decreased to a normal level, but only 9 months if plasma CEA failed to decrease to a normal concentration. During the clinical course of 77% of the patients plasma CEA increased before there was any clinical evidence of recurrence. Plasma CEA levels above 6 ng/ml for nonsmokers and 10 ng/ml for smokers were considered abnormal.

Results of chemotherapy treatment can be predicted with some success by serum CEA levels (Krieger et al., 1983). Serum CEA levels decreased to 30% of the pretreatment CEA values in 30 (57%) of 53 patients studied. Among these 30 patients, 12 had remissions, 15 had no changes, and 3 had progression of the tumor. On the other hand, among 23 patients with unchanged or increasing serum CEA within the first 8 weeks after the initiation of chemotherapy, 19 had progression, 3 no change, and only 1 remission of the tumor. As a result of tumor cell necrosis during therapy there may be a temporary increased release of AFP in the serum and a resultant elevated concentration.

In contrast to this finding, some decrease of serum CEA during chemotherapy may be due to suppressed release from the tumor cells (Kiang and Greenberg, 1983). This inhibition of release was observed in cultured breast carcinoma cells. In 6 patients refractory to previous chemotherapy, serum CEA decreased from 21% to 81% as a result of subsequent treatment. However, during the weeks without chemotherapy, the serum CEA increased again and no clinical response was observed.

A modified homeostatic autoregressive time series model was used by Winkel et al. (1982) in applying serum CEA determinations to 26 postmenopausal breast carcinoma patients during follow-up. Four recurrences without false-positive values were detected by use of this model. It was the most effective approach for detecting recurrences.

In another study CEA in the tissues had no prognostic value as determined by the immunoperoxidase method (Smith et al., 1982). However, CEA in axillary lymph node metastases reflected prognosis. In a group with good prognosis CEA was strongly positive in 24% of all so analyzed. A group (18% of all cases) with weakly positive CEA was associated with poor prognosis, but chemotherapy produced improvement. In the third group (58%) of all cases) CEA was not detected in lymph node metastases, the prognosis was poor, and there was no benefit from chemotherapy.

When two markers—CEA and tissue polypeptide antigen (TPA)—were measured in sera of breast carcinoma patients, one or the other marker was elevated in 95% of the cases (Lüthgens and Schlegel, 1981). Histochemically CEA was demonstrated in all 32 breast carcinoma cases examined by Björklund et al. (1982). With one exception TPA was present also in these cases. With normal values for CEA (5 ng/ml) and TPA (120 U/liter) these markers have proved to be equally suitable in follow-up (Caffier and Brandau, 1983). CEA was more adequate for bone metastases and TPA for visceral involvement.

It is important to consider the possibility that elevated serum CEA values may reflect, besides CEA, the nonspecific cross-reacting antigen (NCA). Polyclonal antibodies to CEA may contain entities reacting with NCA. Therefore, monoclonal antibodies to CEA reflect the actual levels of CEA in the sera or tumor tissues (Nap et al., 1984).

Placental Protein 10 (PP10)

Among the oncofetal markers placental protein 10 (PP10) stands out as the one most frequently associated with breast carcinomas. It was elevated in the serum at a rate of 87% of patients with breast carcinoma (Wurz et al., 1983). It occurred also at abnormally high concentration in the serum of all primary genital tumor patients examined.

Serum Human Chorionic Gonadotropin (HCG)

Serum HCG was elevated in 21% of breast cancer patients (Vaitukaitis et al., 1976), and AFP in 59% (Dash et al., 1979). Since a cross-reactivity between HCG and HLH (human luteinizing hormone) in serum was observed and since there was no evidence of immunohistochemically demonstrable HCG in breast carcinoma tissues (Monteiro et al., 1984), it would appear that what was measured as serum HCG in breast carcinoma patients (Vaitukaitis et al., 1976) actually represented HLH. Therefore it is questionable whether in some breast carcinoma patients with no other marker such measurements still could be of clinical value during follow-up.

CEA-Related Marker (BCGP)

A glycoprotein (BCGP) isolated from a breast carcinoma differed from CEA in the pattern of polyacrylamide gel electrophoresis and immunoelectrophoresis (Kuo et al., 1973). It is related to CEA antigenically, sharing determinants. Antiserum to CEA cross-reacted with BCGP, but after absorption with BCGP the antiserum had only anti-CEA activity. Thus, elevated CEA activities in the sera of patients with breast carcinoma as measured by radioimmunoassay can be related to cross-reactivity with BCGP.

Blood Group M and N Precursor

A delayed-type hypersensitivity reaction to this antigen has been demonstrated regularly in patients with breast carcinoma (Springer, 1984). Delayed-type hypersensitivity response to erythrocyte-derived T antigen has been observed in 89% of 108 ductal carcinoma patients. When normal breast tissues were treated with sialic acid, the T antigen also became unmasked. Whereas in benign lesions it was localized along the luminal cytoplasmic membrane, in cancer cells it was distributed diffusely in the cytoplasm.

Tumor-Associated Markers

There is evidence that breast carcinoma expresses certain substances more frequently than noncancerous tissues. By means of the leukocyte migration technique with carcinoma extracts (Cochran et al., 1974) or leukocyte adherence inhibition microassasy with a carcinoma cell line MCF-7 (Rudczinsky et al., 1978), it was possible to discriminate between cancer patients and controls. The sera of breast carcinoma patients contained antibodies associated with breast carcinoma antigens more frequently than did the sera of patients with other malignancies, those of normal individuals (Gorsky et al., 1976), or those of patients with benign fibrocystic disease (Humphrey et al., 1974). The relative frequency of autoantibodies cross-reacting with carcinoma cells and cells of fibrocystic disease may indicate that there are similar tumor-associated antigens (Sheikh et al., 1976). Breast carcinoma-associated antigen was demonstrated also with a heterologous antiserum to an extract of a duct cell carcinoma (Lerner et al., 1978).

The relationship of these breast carcinoma antigens to embryonal tissues has not been studied.

Lipid-Associated Sialic Acid

A universal tumor-associated marker—lipid-associated sialic acid (LSA)—has elevated serum levels above the normal value of 20 mg% in 86% of breast carcinoma patients (Katopodis et al., 1983). This frequency was observed when the blood samples were examined immediately. If there was a delay, the LSA levels decreased at a rate of 1% per hour, thus decreasing the sensitivity of the marker.

LSA measurements were useful in identifying cases resistent to therapy (Dnistrian et al., 1982). LSA concentration decreased during chemotherapy and remained at low levels in patients without recurrences. LSA increased in 62% of 61 patients with recurrences.

Retinoic Acid-Binding Protein (cRABP)

This protein is present in the normal human uterus and also in breast carcinoma (Huber et al., 1978). It was present in cancer tissues in 52% of 29 cases examined, but not in 32 cases with fibrocystic disease without intraductal epithelial proliferation. When proliferation was present, 6 of 14 cases had cRABP. These findings indicate that proliferative lesions may be closely related to breast carcinomas.

Cellular Protein p53

This is a cell protein in a complex with SV40 large T-antigen in SV40-transformed mouse cells. p53 is present also in nontransformed cells. In a screening of 155 breast cancer patients for the presence of autoantibodies to p53, 10% proved to have anti-p53 activity, whereas none of the 164 control women had evidence of such antibodies (Crawford et al., 1982). The immunological response to p53 of breast cancer patients can be either the altered structure of this antigen or production in excessive amounts. It is possible that other malignant neoplasms elicit a similar reaction.

Phosphohexose Isomerase

This enzyme has proved useful in monitoring patients treated with chemotherapy (Leroux et al., 1978). It increased when breast carcinoma metastasized to liver or bone and decreased in response to therapy.

5′-Nucleotide Phosphodiesterase Isoenzyme V (5′-NPD-V)

Elevated serum levels of 5′-NPD-V were found in 86% of patients with breast carcinomas metastatic to the liver and with abnormal liver scans (Tsou et al., 1982a). In the absence of other liver function abnormalities, 29% of 41 such patients had elevated 5′NPD-V. The elevation of this enzyme may be due not to its increased synthesis by tumor cells but to the presence of more cells in liver cell regeneration.

The Creatine Kinase Isoenzyme CPK-BB

Serum levels of brain creatine kinase-BB were found to be elevated above 3 ng/ml in 80% of patients with metastatic breast carcinoma and 60% with local disease in a study by Thompson et al. (1980). The normal range was reported 0.5–3.7 ng/ml. Measurement of CPK-BB was a useful indicator of the response to treatment.

Ferritin

Daliford et al (1984) reported that the clinical course of breast cancer was reflected in serum ferritin levels in 77% of their patients during follow-up. However, elevated serum ferritin concentration can occur with diseases other than malignant neoplasms. False-positive values were observed with a frequency of 23%.

Immunohistochemically very little ferritin was seen in tumor cells in a study by Rossiello et al (1984). Most of it was in the histiocytes and connective tissue stroma. Therefore, increased serum ferritin concentrations may not only be derived from the tumor cells but may be a result of stromal reaction. In 40% of 20 carcinoma cases tumor cells contained transferrin, Lactoferrin was present only in normal epithelial cells and benign lesions.

The appearance of ferritin-bearing lymphocytes in peripheral blood may mark the recurrence of the breast carcinoma (Moroz et al., 1984). In some patients with carcinoma and premalignant lesions the test was positive while there was no evidence of breast disease by physical examination and mammography.

Urinary Androgen Metabolites

Androsterone and etiocholanolone are tumor-associated markers differing from all others by their decrease rather than increase as indicator of poor prognosis. When the urinary values of these androgen metabolites were below the median amount, the recurrence of early breast carcinomas has been found to be more frequent than in those patients with the steroid values above the median amount (Thomas et al., 1982). This relationship was more pronounced in pre- than in postmenopausal women.

Polyamines

Polyamine excretion in urine was increased in 65% of 34 breast carcinoma patients studied by Romano et al. (1983). Putrescine excretion was associated more frequently with bone and visceral metastases, while spermidine and spermine were associated with visceral metastases only. Polyamine levels have been found to correlate with metastatic spead to various organs (Chayen et al., 1983). There was not such correlation of spermine with lymph node metastases (Chayen et al., 1983), tumor size, or histologic appearance. Putrescine, spermidine, and spermine levels in carcinoma tissues have been found to reflect prognosis (Kingsnorth et al., 1984). Recurrences within two years after mastectomy were associated with high polyamine levels in the tissues.

Breast Tissue-Associated Antigens

Levels of antibody complexes with M_r 85,000 antigen were significantly higher in the sera of breast cancer patients studied by Koestler et al. (1981) than in the sera of controls.

Another human breast tissue-associated antigen was detected by a monoclonal antibody to human breast carcinoma cell line MCF-7 (Thompson et al., 1983b). This M_r 100,000 antigen was present in 92% of 13 breast carcinoma tissues, in gynecomastic epithelium, and in lesser amounts in normal breast epithelium when evaluated immunohistochemically. Although noticeable in small amounts in normal tissues, it was present in significantly increased amounts in the sera of breast cancer patients.

A human IgM monoclonal antibody was produced by fusion of human lymphocytes from a lymph node of a breast carcinoma patient with a murine myeloma cell line, which was not secreting immunoglobulin (Teramato et al., 1982). This antibody reacted with 81% of 67 tissue samples of primary breast carcinomas, all of 20 samples of metastases, and 14% of 22 samples of benign breast lesions.

Cells With High-Avidity Fc Receptors

Such peripheral blood mononuclear cells (T or null cells) were found to be significantly more numerous in patients with breast carcinoma than in controls (Bray and McPherson, 1981). The incidence of such cells correlated with tumor burden was usable as a marker to evaluate clinical condition.

α-Lactalbumin

This is a milk protein. It was demonstrated immunohistochemically by Lee et al. (1984) in 6% of breast carcinomas and in 62% of the metastases in various sites. The specificity of the reaction demonstrating the α-lactalbumin was established by absorption of the polyclonal antibodies with the antigen. Although cross-reacting antigens were present in other tumors, such as mesotheliomas and salivary gland and skin appendage tumors, α-lactalbumin was a suitable marker for breast carcinomas, especially when it was necessary to identify a tumor from unknown sources.

Tumor-Specific Markers

The presence of specific markers in breast carcinoma tissues has been suggested by lymphocyte cytotoxicity microassay (Fossati et al., 1972), delayed hypersensitivity skin reactions (Hollinshead et al., 1974), leukocyte migration inhibition assay (McCoy et al., 1976), transfer factor assay (Byers et al., 1976), autologous antibody and heterologous antisera studies (Fett et al., 1978), and immunoperoxidase microscopy (Yu et al., 1980), and by raising monoclonal antibodies by the fusion of human lymphocytes from breast cancer patients' lymph nodes with murine nonproducer myeloma cells (Schlom et al., 1980). Evaluating T-lymphocyte-mediated immune responsiveness, Munther et al. (1980) showed that cystosarcoma phyllodes and adenocarcinoma of the breast shared a tumor-specific antigen. In these studies, breast carcinoma antigen was limited to breast tissues.

Evidence of a specific breast carcinoma component has been produced by the leukocyte adherence inhibition assay. All 17 breast carcinoma cases studied by Tsang et al. (1982) were correctly identified by a positive reaction. None of the 20 normal individuals or 10 with benign breast disease had a positive reaction.

The presence of specific antigen was also demonstrated with monoclonal antibodies (Kufe et al., 1983). These antibodies lysed mammary tumor cells in an antibody-dependent cell-mediated cytotoxicity reaction. They reacted with mammary tumor cells from 4 of 6 pleural effusions.

In our investigations (Berkman et al., 1975) using appropriately absorbed rabbit immune serum to breast carcinoma, we observed a cross-reacting antigen shared by breast carcinomas and other tumors. The specific peroxidase staining was most striking in breast carcinomas.

A Nuclear Antigen

Using a specific antiserum in the complement fixation method, Chiu et al. (1977) demonstrated that there was a specific antigen in breast carcinoma dehistonized chromatin. This antiserum did not react with other tumors or placenta.

β_2-Microglobulin-Associated Antigen

Breast carcinoma-specific antigen was demonstrated in tumor tissues by Thomson et al. (1978). It had a molecular weight within a range of 70,000–150,000 and consisted of subunits, the most prominent of which had molecular weights of 40,000, 25,000, and 12,000. This antigen was immunologically related to HLA antigens and was associated with β_2-microglobulin. It is possible that similar antigens were synthesized by a human mammary carcinoma cell line BT20 (Hurlimann and Dayal, 1978).

Breast Carcinoma-Specific Glycoproteins

Three groups of investigators have reported specific breast carcinoma glycoproteins with molecular weights from 52,700 to 67,000 (Holton et al., 1980; Kamiyama et al., 1980; Leung et al., 1981). It is possible that these antigens constitute one entity or are closely related.

One of them was present in the plasma membrane of the tumor cells (Leung et al., 1981). It has a molecular weight of 52,700 and α_2-electrophoretic mobility. Related to this, a cytosol mammary tumor glycoprotein (MTGP) was isolated on the basis of physicochemical properties from one primary and one metastatic breast carcinoma (Sundblat and Edgington, 1983). The molecular weight of MTGP was found to be 20,000 by exclusion chromatography and 40,000 by sodium dodecyl sulfate polyacrylamide gel electrophoresis.

Antigens were isolated from immune complexes (Maidment et al., 1981) with a molecular weight of 20,000–42,000 and isoelectric points between pH 3.0 and 5.0. They were not further defined, but they may be specific in breast carcinomas.

Antibodies generated by fusion of lymphocytes from a lymph node with metastic breast carcinoma to mouse myeloma cells reacted with 40–60% malignant cells (Imam et al., 1983). Although corresponding antigen has not been defined, such specific human antibodies may be more valuable in future use not only for monitoring patients with malignant disease, but also for therapy being less likely to cause undesirable reactions associated with heterologous immunoglobulins.

Using four monoclonal antibodies to mammary tumor cells, Hand et al (1983) observed different patterns and reactivity in breast carcinomas. This phenotypic variation, as defined by monoclonal antibodies, was observed even in single-cell clones.

Components of Mouse Mammary Tumor Virus (MMTV)

Lopez et al (1981) reported that MMTV induced an enhanced lymphoproliferative response in a peripheral T-cell subset of breast cancer patients. This subset was characterized as E-rosetting, Leu-1-positive, and surface immunoglobulin-negative. By the leukocyte migration inhibition test it has been shown that breast cancer patients have a high frequency of response to MMTV (Fukuda, 1980b), but not to Mason-Pfizer virus or mouse leukemia virus. It has been shown that there are unique RNA sequences in breast carcinoma that are homologous to RNA of MMTV (Axel et al., 1972a). Seventy percent of adenocarcinoma tissues were able to synthesize particles containing RNA-instructed DNA polymerase (Axel et al., 1972b). Subsequently, an antigen related to gp52 of the MMTV was seen in 39% of 131 female breast carcinomas (Mesa-Tejada et al., 1978) and in 89% of 36 male breast carcinomas (Lloyd et al., 1982). Using an immunohistochemical approach they located gp52 in lymph node tumors, and primary breast carcinoma was suggested. Subsequently, the primary breast carcinoma containing gp52 was found. More recently particles resembling retroviruses were detected in some clonal derivatives of the human breast carcinoma cell line T47D (Keydar et al., 1984). These particles and the cultured media contained an antigen cross-reacting with the antibodies to gp52 of the MMTV.

Circulating antibodies to MMTV were detected in 40% of 148 patients with breast cancer, in 5 of 27 with benign breast diseases, in 7 of 60 with other malignancies, and in 2 of 56 without history of previous cancer (Tomana et al., 1981a). Such antibodies were present more frequently in older breast cancer patients. A higher incidence of MMTV-associated antigen was detected in another series of studies (Holder and Hells, 1983). An antiserum to MMTV reacted with 86% of sera from 68 patients with breast cancer, 13% of sera from 61 normal controls or patients with benign breast diseases, and 11% of 18 with other malignant neoplasms. Similar incidences of reactivity were observed in tissues. While MMTV blocked the reaction of antibody with the carcinoma tissues, p52 of MMTV did not. The nature of the antigen and the significance of it in normal individuals is not known.

The latter findings do not indicate that human breast carcinoma tissues produce gene products identical to those of the MMTV. We have shown cross-reactivity between human cytotrophoblasts and MMTV (Klavins et al., 1980). On the other hand, there is evidence that normal human cells contain DNA sequences related to MMTV (Callahan et al., 1982). Thus, the expression of a breast carcinoma antigen related to MMTV could be the expression of an oncofetal gene product. Antibodies cross-reacting with mouse mammary tumors have been detected in some healthy women (Tomana et al., 1981b). It is therefore possible that human and MMTV genomes have some sequences for the synthesis of immunologically similar, not necessarily identical, gene products. A human milk protein is immunologically related to gp55, the major envelope glycoprotein of MMTV (Dion et al., 1980). This was shown with micro-Ouchterlony immunodiffusion assay. The human fraction was a glycoprotein with a molecular weight of 58,000. Other similarities were the same NH_2-terminus for two common peptides of human milk protein and MMTV gp55 or gp50. It has also been suggested (Zotter et al., 1981) that there is a human virus similar to MMTV.

From transfection of NIH 3T3 mouse cells with DNA from MMTV-induced tumors, chemically induced mouse breast tumors, and human mammary carcinoma cell line MCF-7, it appeared that identical or closely related transforming genes were activated in these tumors (Lane et al., 1981). The transforming activities of the DNA of all these tumors were inactivated by restriction endonucleases PvuII and SACI, but not by BamHI, EcoRI, HindIII, KpnI, or XhoI.

A glycoprotein with a molecular weight of 86,000 is an antigen that has been specifically associated with the expression of the transforming genes of both human and mouse mammary carcinomas (Becker et al., 1982).

Certain DNA sequences of MMTV were shown to be homologous with the EcoRI DNA fragment of tumors among 28 examined (Crepin et al., 1984). MMTV-related sequences were also present in the lymphocytes of these patients.

Rous Sarcoma Virus-Related pp60c-src

An increased pp60c-*src* protein kinase activity (4- to 20-fold) compared with normal tissues was present in 7 of 20 human mammary carcinomas studied by Jacobs and Rubsamen (1983). The patients with such tumors had no detectable antibodies against cellular or viral pp60-*src*. As in other neoplasms, this is an example of augmented oncogene expression, which may be related to carcinogenesis. The excess of cellular oncogene product may serve as a tumor marker.

Paget's Disease

Using the gross cystic disease fluid protein GCDFP-15, a marker of breast dysplasias, Mazoujian et al. (1984) established that extramammary Paget's disease is derived from apocrine cells. Antibodies to GCDFP-15 were localized in 6 of 7 cases including 5 from vulva and 1 from the axilla. As expected, since GCDFP is a marker for apocrine cells, it was localized only in apocrine ducts and glands of normal skin. CEA also was present in all seven cases.

Serum CEA was elevated in 3 of 10 patients with genital Paget's disease studied by Oji et al. (1984). These three patients had widespread metastases. Serum CEA was not increased above normal values in 7 patients with more localized disease.

In another study (Kariniemi et al., 1984), CEA was found in all 12 extramammary and in 5 of 7 mammary Paget disease tumors studied. Along with CEA there was also the apocrine epithelial antigen. Both these markers were present also in the intraductal or ductal carcinomas associated with mammary Paget's disease. Thus all these entities apparently have a common origin from sweat gland ducts with an apocrine differentiation.

BRAIN TUMORS

Oncofetal Markers

CEA concentration in serum and cyst fluid correlated with the degree of malignancy of the gliomas studied by Hill and Hunt (1982). CEA values were elevated also in acoustic neuromas, craniopharyngiomas, and colloid or hemorrhagic cysts.

Fetal brain contains antigens, such as OFA (Irie et al., 1976), that may cross-react with a wide variety of malignant neoplasms. In addition, there are gene products with a more restricted cross-reactivity, limited to brain tumors. Four monoclonal antibodies, raised to second-trimester human fetal brain tissue, reacted predominantly with glioblastoma cell lines and also with cell lines of neuroblastomas and melanomas (Wikstrand and Bigner, 1982; Wikstrand et al., 1982).

Neuroblastomas

Oncofetal Neuroblastoma Antigens

Spleen cells of mice immunized with human neuroblastoma and hybridized with a mouse plasmacytoma produced antibodies reacting specifically with all human neuroblastomas tested and with fetal brain (Kennett and Gilbert, 1979). In addition, these antibodies reacted with a retinoblastoma and a glioiblastoma. Elevated serum CEA was present in 35% of patients with neuroblastomas (Helson et al., 1976).

With a rabbit antiserum to first-trimester fetal brain, two antigens were detected on neuroblastoma cells (Danon et al., 1980). One antigen was cross-reacting with the first-trimester brain, neuroblastoma, and other tumor cells; the other antigen cross-reacted only with the fetal brain and neuroblastoma cells.

Tumor-Associated Markers

Ferritin

Ferritin estimation in serum has served as an indicator of prognosis in children with stage IV neuroblastomas (Hann et al., 1983). With serum ferritin levels less than 150 ng/ml the probability of 2-year progression-free survival was 27% of 52 patients, but only 2.3% of 89 patients with serum ferritin levels greater than 151 ng/ml. In females corresponding values were 47% survival of 19 with lower levels and 3% survival of 39 with higher levels; and 75% of patients less than 1 year of age with low ferritin levels experienced 2 years progression-free survival, while none of 9 with a high concentration of serum ferritin had such survival.

γ-γ-enolase

γ-γ-enolase (NSE) is a sensitive marker for neuroblastomas. It is specific to nervous system tissues. Ishiguro et al. (1982) found this enolase to range from 13.6 to 33.0 ng/ml, 20–30 times higher than in controls, in the serum of neuroblastoma patients with the exception of ganglioneuroblastoma patients, who had no elevated serum enolase. In a study by Zeiter et al. (1983), serum levels greater than 100 ng/ml were associated with poor prognosis, especially in children below 1 year of age. All 7 children with NSE less than

100 ng/ml were alive 3 years after the initial diagnosis, whereas 7 of 8 with NSE greater than 100 ng/ml died within 1 year.

NSE can also be demonstrated immunohistochemically in all neuroblastomas (Tsokos et al., 1984). Morphologically similar tumors, such as Ewing sarcomas, lymphomas, and other soft tissue tumors, did not contain demonstrable NSE. NSE was present in differentiated myoblasts of an embryonal rhabdomyosarcoma.

Neuroblastoma-Specific Membrane Antigens

Antisera in rabbits and a monkey were raised with neuroblastoma tissues by Raney et al. (1978). After appropriate absorption, these antisera reacted with neuroblastoma cells and the reactivity, as expressed by complement-dependent microcytotoxicity, was not abolished by absorption with normal monkey or rabbit brain tissues.

*Amplification of N-*myc *Oncogene*

As in other malignant neoplasms, neuroblastomas too are associated with oncogene amplification. Of 63 untreated patients studied by Brodeur et al. (1984), 38% had neuroblastomas with 3- to 100-fold amplification of the N-*myc*. The degree of amplification correlated with the advancement of the disease. There was no evidence of N-*myc* amplification in stages 1 and 2.

Gliomas

Oncofetal Glioma Antigens

Surface antigens of glioma cells were shown to cross-react with antigens of fetal brain by Wikstrand and Bigner (1979). Heterologous antiserum (Kehayov, 1976) appropriately absorbed and autologous immune serum (Trouillas, 1971) to gliomas cross-reacted with fetal brain. Using monoclonal antibodies to human fetal brain, Wikstrand et al (1981) found that human fetal brain contains antigens cross-reacting with human glioblastoma cells and some tumor cells derived from neural crest.

Glioma-Specific Antigens

Using rabbit antiserum to human gliomas, Mahaley (1971) suggested that there might be specific antigens. Such specific antigens were present on membranes of established cell lines from gliomas studied by Wahlstrom et al. (1974). Apparently, low-molecular-weight components are unique in glioblastoma cells (Hitchcock et al., 1979). Furthermore, glioma-specific antigens are shared, as shown by heteroantiserum cytotoxicity (Coakham and Lakshmi, 1975; Wikstrand et al., 1977) and autoantibody (Sheikh et al.,

1977) studies. Some of the glioma antigens are also shared with melanomas (Pfreundschuh et al., 1978). Common glioma membrane antigens were not detected in fetal or adult brain or other tissues by Birkmayer and Stass (1980).

Among several monoclonal antibodies to a glioma cell line there was one (MCA 2F3) that recognized a specific antigen in 9 of 11 glioblastoma tissues (Wikstrand et al., 1984). This antibody did not react with other normal or neoplastic tissues.

Virus-Related Components

In a study by Cuatico et al. (1973), gliomas were shown to contain particles partly made up of 70S RNA and RNA-directed DNA polymerase. These entities were not found in normal tissues or known RNA viruses. They were less frequently observed in ependymomas, menigiomas, and Schwannomas. Electron microscopically these particles looked similar to C-type RNA viruses (Birkmayer et al., 1974a). One of 6 astrocytomas in short-term cultures produced RNA particles with incomplete retrovirus characteristics (Thorne et al., 1982).

Medulloblastomas

Oncofetal Medulloblastoma Antigens

These antigens are shared by human fetal brain and medulloblastomas. Using immunodiffusion and immunoelectrophoresis methods Kehayov et al. (1979) detected them in the cerebrospinal fluid of patients with medulloblastoma but not in their serum.

Medulloblastoma-Specific Antigen

Medulloblastoma-specific antigen was detected by Sato et al. (1978) with a rabbit antiserum to medulloblastoma cells. There was not cross-reactivity of this antigen with other brain tumors.

RNA Particles

Thorne et al. (1982) reported that, after short-term culturing of medulloblastoma cells, 4 of 7 such tumors released RNA particles. They resembled an incomplete retrovirus.

Meningiomas

Oncofetal Meningioma Antigen

This antigen is shared by human embryonic brain of 8–10 weeks gestation and meningiomas according to Kehayov et al. (1976).

Meningioma-Specific Antigens

Serologic studies by Catalano et al. (1972) and Winters and Rich (1975) have indicated the presence of specific antigens in meningiomas. An antigen has been isolated in a chromatographically pure form (Kehayov et al., 1977).

SV40-Related Antigens in Meningiomas

Three of eight meningiomas tested by Weiss et al., (1975) contained T and U antigens related to Simian sarcomavirus 40. There was also a typical loss of G-22 chromosome as it occurs in SV40-transformed cells. Zimmermann et al. (1981) reported that anti-SV40 sera reacted with 3 of 5 human meningioma cell lines in tissue culture. These cells did not express viral capsid (V) antigen. By electron microscopy Weiss et al. (1976) observed particles resembling Papovaviruses.

Ependymal Tumors: SV40-Related Antigens

An antigen related to T antigen of SV40 was demonstrated with immunoperoxidase microscopy (Tabuchi et al., 1978). This antigen was localized in the nuclei of a choroid plexus papilloma and an ependymoma. It was not present in 37 other different brain tumors examined. It may well be a significant association even though only two tumors of ependymal origin have been examined. It is known that in Papovaviruse-induced brain tumors in hamsters there is predominance of such ependyma-derived neoplasms.

RETINOBLASTOMAS

Elevated serum levels of both AFP and CEA are present in 80% of patients with retinoblastomas (Michelson et al., 1976). In children, the normal values of serum CEA were found to be 1.04 $\pm$ 0.42 ng/ml and AFP 8.71 $\pm$ 4.46 ng/ml (Minei et al., 1983). Both these markers were elevated in the serum of 4 of 13 patients before the treatment. They returned to normal levels after treatment. Caution should be exercised regarding the use of CEA as a marker for this type of malignant neoplasm. There was no histochemically demonstrable CEA, using immunoperoxidase method, in any of the 47 retinoblastoma cases examined by Kivela and Tarkkanen (1983). It is not known why elevated serum CEA levels are associated with this neoplasm. CEA values in aqueous humor and subretinal fluid were found to be lower than those in serum (Das et al., 1984).

Retinoblastoma-Specific Markers

Immune complexes have been studied in patients with retinoblastomas. The antigens were partially characterized by polyacrylamide gel electrophoresis. They might represent tumor-specific or idiotypic antigens (Stein et al., 1980a). There is 10-fold to 200-fold amplification of N-*myc* genes in retnoblastomas and cell lines of these tumors as estimated by the high levels of N-*myc* mRNA (Lee et al., 1984). Under similar experimental conditions, there was no N-*myc* gene expression in fibroblasts.

CARCINOMAS OF THE THYROID GLAND

There is evidence that a substance of a molecular weight of approximately 45,000 contains a specific marker for thyroid carcinomas (Aoki and De Groot, 1982). This substance was isolated from a mixed papillary-follicular adenocarcinoma of the thyroid gland. Only patients with thyroid carcinomas had a positive leukocyte migration inhibition reaction when this substance was used in the assay.

Medullary Carcinomas of the Thyroid

Calcitonin

Calcitonin is a most suitable marker for monitoring patients with medullary thyroid carcinoma. It was elevated above normal levels (0.02–0.18 ng/ml) in serum of all 19 patients with this type of thyroid carcinoma studied by Busnardo et al. (1984). After treatment the calcitonin level in the serum decreased. By selective venous catheterization and determination of serum calcitonin, it has been possible to localize tumors and perform effective surgical procedures (Norton et al., 1980).

There are some healthy individuals with high concentrations of plasma calcitonin when measured by immunological methods. The interference of calcitonin-like immunoreactivity can be eliminated by extracting the plasma on columns of silica (Body and Heath, 1984).

CEA

While CEA as a marker is less useful for differentiated carcinomas, it can be used as an effective tumor marker for medullary carcinomas of the thyroid gland. It was elevated in the serum in 84% of the cases of this disease reported by Calmettes et al. (1978). In conjunction with calcitonin these markers were applicable to the diagnosis also.

CEA is present in C cells. It persists throughout the development of medullary carcinoma from the early to later stages, whereas calcitonin may decrease within tumor cells in cases of rapidly growing tumors with metastases (Mendelsohn et al., 1984).

It is possible that certain poorly differentiated follicular carcinomas represent a separate group of thyroid neoplasms. Besides elevated CEA and calcitonin levels in patients' serum these tumors contained both markers in the cells as demonstrated histochemically (Calmettes et al., 1982).

In advanced disease, serum CEA levels may reflect a poor prognosis more accurately than calcitonin (Busnardo et al., 1983). Overall CEA appeared to be a more sensitive marker than calcitonin (Rougier et al., 1983). CEA was a better prognostic indicator for the medullary thyroid carcinomas taking into consideration the slopes of serial CEA determinations (Saad et al, 1984). A steep slope was associated with a rapidly progressing disease and a flat one with no metastases or nonprogressive disease.

Diamine Oxidase

Several investigators have found that serum diamine oxidase activity is markedly elevated in patients with medullary carcinoma of the thyroid gland (Scalabrino and Feroli, 1982). This increased activity originated from the tumor tissues owing to an increased synthesis. Since the activity of diamine oxidase was not increased as frequently as calcitonin in the patients' sera, the latter appeared to be the better marker of the two.

Papillary and Follicular Adenocarcinomas

Elevated serum calcitonin levels have been reported in patients with other carcinomas as well—hepatomas and lung carcinomas (Mulder et al., 1981), especially of the small-cell type (Cuttitta et al., 1981; Krauss et al., 1981; Wallach et al., 1981).

Serum CEA above 10 ng/ml was observed by Madeddu et al. (1980) in 32% of patients with differentiated carcinomas of the thyroid gland. These tumors included papillary, follicular, and mixed papillary-follicular carcinomas. None of the 258 patients with thyroid nodules had serum CEA levels above 12 ng/ml.

The combined procedures of ^{131}I total-body scanning and measurement of serum thyroglobulin have proved effective in detecting recurrences of differentiated carcinomas (Roti et al., 1982).

Hemangioendotheliomas of the Thyroid

The histogenesis of these tumors was resolved by the use of antibodies to factor VIII-related antigen (Schaffer and Ormanns, 1983). The factor VIII-related antigen is a specific marker for endothelial cells. The antibodies reacted in immunohistochemical tests with 4 of 6 such tumors. This finding supports the view that the hemangioendotheliomas of the thyroid gland are not undifferentiated carcinomas of special type but are of endothelial origin.

Immunoradiodiagnosis

Immunoradiodiagnosis using ^{131}I-labeled monoclonal antibodies to CEA has been successful (Berche et al., 1982). With transaxial tomoscintigraphy, after the injection of labeled antibodies, 94% of 17 tumor sites were detected. With conventional scintigraphy the sensitivity was only 43%. These studies included both medullary thyroid carcinomas and gastrointestinal carcinomas.

TUMORS OF THE LARYNX

LDH Isoenzyme—A Tumor-Specific Marker

A unique LDH isoenzyme was found by Tanaka et al. (1976) in the serum of a patient with carcinoma of the larynx. This isoenzyme disappeared after removal of the tumor. It was stable at 57°C for 30 min.

A monoclonal antibody to laryngeal carcinoma cells reacted with two types of laryngeal carcinoma cells and also two types of salivary gland tumor cells but not with normal human cells tested (Zenner, 1981). This indicates the presence of an antigen with some specificity for these tumors.

Viruses in Papillomas

Costa et al. (1981) obtained evidence that human papillomavirus causes juvenile multiple laryngeal papillomas. This was also established by hybridization studies with an *in vitro* labeled bovine papillomavirus type 1 probe and detection of intranuclear group-specific structural antigens (Lancaster and Jenson, 1981). Human papillomavirus (HPV) DNA was found in 12 juvenile-onset and 8 adult-onset laryngeal papillomas (Mounts et al., 1982). The viral DNA was HPV-6 with four subtypes. In addition, HPV capsid antigen was detected in two juvenile onset and two adult-onset papillomas.

Epstein-Barr virus (EBV) nuclear antigen and DNA were found in tumor cells in 3 of 5 patients with supraglottic laryngeal carcinomas (Brichacek et al., 1983). These five patients had antibodies to early antigen of the virus. Like nasopharyngeal carcinomas, these laryngeal tumors may be associated with EBV infection.

LUNG CARCINOMAS

Expression of different tumor markers by different lung carcinomas was studied by establishing 23 tissue-cultured lines from xenografted carcinomas (Shorthouse et al., 1982). ACTH was expressed in 78% (11 small-cell, 2 squamous, 2 large-cell, and 3 adenocarcinomas), CEA in 57% (7 small-cell, 2 squamous, 1 large-cell, 3 adenocarcinomas), β-subunit of HCG in 13% (1 small-cell, 2 large-cell anaplastic, and calcitonin in 13% (2 small-cell and 1 adenocarcinoma) of lung tumors studied.

Oncofetal Markers

Elevated serum CEA was found in 88% of patients with lung carcinomas studied by Barbolin et al (1980). This is one of the highest frequencies of increased CEA concentration reported in various studies.

The oncofetal markers HCG (Kozielski, 1982) and AFP (Waldmann and McIntire, 1974) occurred at elevated levels only in 44% and 7% of lung cancer patients, respectively. As expected, the tissue concentration of various markers is higher than that in the serum. CEA was present in 71% of 101 tumors and β-HCG was present in 36% of 97 lung carcinomas examined immunohistochemically by Harach et al. (1983).

CEA

With 10 ng/ml as an upper limit of normal serum concentration of CEA for patients without lung tumors, the incidence of elevated CEA in 50 lung carcinoma patients reported by Mondagini et al. (1982) was only 30%. In all investigations the sensitivity depends on the upper limit of normal values. When the β_2-microglobulin was estimated concomitantly, 48% of patients had increased serum concentration of one or the other marker. Serum CEA above 10 ng/ml was an indicator of the most unvavorable prognosis, according to Dobrovolskii et al. (1983). The amount of CEA in serum correlated with the survival time of the patients and the effectiveness of treatment.

These high CEA values correlated with the nuclear DNA pattern (Ozaki et al., 1982). Triploid or mixed-type nuclear DNA was associated with plasma CEA levels greater than 15.0 ng/ml. This was not so with diploid-tetraploid type.

It may be possible to detect early-developing carcinomas by histochemical examination of the exfoliated cells for the presence of CEA (Boon et al., 1982). Not only tumor cells but some morphologically benign squamous epithelial cells have been found to contain CEA. Such CEA-containing squamous cells were present in the sputum of high-risk patients without clinical evidence of carcinoma. In another immunohistochemical study CEA was demonstrated in 71% of 101 tumors (Harach et al., 1983).

Among 17 patients with pleural malignancy-associated fluids, 65% had CEA values of 4–60 ng/ml in these effusions (Heyenga and Morr, 1982). There was no elevated CEA concentration (0–2 ng/ml) in the fluids associated with disease other than malignant neoplasms. CEA determination of pleural fluids of suspected malignancy can complement cytological examination in the diagnosis.

The highest CEA concentration was associated with adenocarcinomas in a study by Tourine and Deschamps (1982). There was a variation of sensitivity and specificity depending on the set values. At a 5 ng/ml or greater value the specificity was 100%, but the sensitivity only 53% (Prigogine et al., 1982).

T Antigen

T antigen, the precursor of blood group MN antigens, was used to test the intradermal delayed hypersensitivity reaction of lung carcinoma patients. Of 87, 90% had a positive reaction, whereas all 85 healthy persons and 94% of patients with benign lung disease had a negative reaction (Springer, 1984).

Ferritin-like Fetal Protein

This marker was isolated from a squamous cell carcinoma of the lung (Satoh et al., 1975). It is an iron-containing protein with molecular weight of 180,000, thus differing from α_2-HF (Buffe and Rimbaut, 1975), which has 600,000 molecular weight. The isoelectric point of this protein is 5.5 and on SDS gel electrophoresis it yields subunits with a molecular weight of 20,000. Although there has been no direct comparison, it is possible that this ferritin-like protein is similar to an antigen (LTFA) isolated from lung tumor and fetal lung extracts (Sega et al., 1980).

Antigens in Bronchogenic Carcinomas

An antiserum to an adenocarcinoma of the lung has been shown to cross-react with squamous cell carcinomas of lung and fetal lung tissue extracts (Bell, 1976). Significantly less of this antigen was present in oat cell carcinomas and normal adult tissues with the exception of lung. This antigen differed from AFP, CEA, and blood group substances.

Using a similar approach with a squamous cell carcinoma as the antigenic source (Kelly and Levy, 1977) and with an oat cell carcinoma as the antigen (Ford and Newman, 1979), the investigators demonstrated the presence of cross-reacting oncofetal antigen in different lung tumors. It was not present in adult normal lung tissues. When a radioimmunoassay was used to evaluate the presence of an oncofetal antigen with a molecular weight of approximately 32,000, it was found in all types of human lung tumors (Kempner et al., 1979). In addition, some colon, prostate, and breast tumors and normal brain had evidence of this antigen.

Tumor-Associated Markers

Calcitonin

Measurement of serum calcitonin concentration has been clinically useful in treating patients with lung carcinomas (Krauss et al., 1981; Wallach et al.,

1981). Serum calcitonin was found to be elevated in about 54% of 41 bronchogenic carcinomas (Tabolli et al., 1983). Among 194 lung carcinoma patients examined by Luster et al. (1982), increased serum calcitonin levels were found in 57% with small-cell carcinoma, in 10% with squamous cell carcinoma, and in only 2 patients with large-cell carcinoma. Together with CEA, calcitonin determinations may increase the probablity of detecting a marker for follow-up of lung carcinoma patients.

HNT

The glycopeptide HNT is a well-characterized tumor-associated marker for carcinomas of the lung (Chan, JS, et al., 1983). The amino-terminal portion with the 76 amino acids of pro-opiomelanocortin constitute the peptide of HNT. It was present in the plasma of normal individuals without pituitary dysfunction in amounts less than 100 pg/mi. Of 30 patients with squamous cell carcinoma 47% had plasma HNT values greater than 100 pg/ml; and 74% of 35 patients with small-cell carcinoma had such an increase of plasma HNT. Elevated plasma HNT was noted also in 2 of 8 patients with adenocarcinoma, 2 of 4 with large-cell undifferentiated carcinoma, and both of 2 with carcinoid tumors. The overall frequency of elevated plasma HNT levels in patients with pulmonary cancers was 60%. Plasma HNT above 100 pg/ml was also observed in 25% of 20 patients with pulmonary diseases other than malignant neoplasms. As expected, the HNT concentration in pulmonary venous blood was 16–86% higher than the pulmonary arterial blood measured in 8 patients with carcinomas at the time of surgery.

An antigen with a molecular weight of approximately 40,000 has been isolated from a bronchogenic carcinoma (Frost et al., 1975). It was heat-stable at 50°C for 30 min and migrated with a cationic mobility on immunoelectrophoresis at a pH of 8.5. This antigen was present in normal lung tissues also, but in significantly smaller quantities than in adenocarcinomas or squamous cell carcinomas of the lung.

Monoclonal antibodies have been produced by a cell line (NCI-H69) from a small-cell carcinoma of the lung (Cuttitta et al., 1981) These antibodies were relatively specific for small-cell, squamous, and adenocarcinomas of the lung. They reacted also with neuroblastomas and breast cancer and insignificantly with normal human adult tissues. To measure another lung carcinoma-associated antigen the RIA method was developed (Braatz et al., 1983). The normal value was considered to be 0.92 $\pm$ 0.43 SD μg/ml. Values greater than 2 SD above normal were considered positive. The frequencies of positive sera among different patients were the following: for pulmonary squamous cell carcinoma 42% of 31, for adenocarcinoma 60% of

15, for large-cell carcinoma 17% of 18, for small-cell carcinoma 19% of 16, and for other carcinomas 13% of 23. The false-positive rate was 2% of 88 controls. It appeared useful in early detection and monitoring of the disease process. Subsequently the enzyme-linked immunosorbent assay (ELISA) appeared to be ten times more sensitive than the RIA method and five times more efficient in antigen utilization (Hua et al., 1984).

Pregnancy-associated α-2-glycoprotein was found to be present in the sera of patients with lung cancer at a rate of 81% (Watanabe, 1980). It was not useful as a marker, but did serve as an indicator of the course of the disease. In this respect, measurement of serum calcitonin levels was also useful (Krauss et al., 1981; Wallach et al., 1981). The highest levels of calcitonin were in sera of patients with small-cell carcinoma.

Surfactant-Associated Proteins in Alveolar Cell Carcinomas

Espinoza et al. (1982) were able to differentiate alveolar cell carcinomas from other lung tumors by the presence of surfactant-associated proteins in tumor cells with alveolar cell differentiation. Such proteins were not present in the other kinds of lung tumors.

Frossman Antigen Synthesis and Degradation Enzymes in Squamous Cell Carcinomas

Activity of UDP-acetyl-galactosaminogloboside-alpha-N-acetylgalactosaminyltransferase and alpha-N-acetyl-D-galactosaminidase were consistently elevated in squamous cell carcinoma compared with noninvolved lung tissues in studies by Taniguchi et al (1981). Such consistency was not observed in adenocarcinomas, although the mean enzyme activities were higher than in uninvolved lung tissues.

Serum Protein-Bound Carbohydrates in Small-Cell Carcinomas

Waalkes et al. (1983) found that serum protein-bound fucose was elevated at a frequency of 92.5% and mannose and galactose at 77.5% of 40 patients with small-cell carcinomas of the lung. In 95% of the patients the serum prior to treatment contained elevated levels of at least one of these protein-bound neutral carbohydrates. A biomarker index was calculated as a summation of all three sugar levels. This index correlated with the tumor burden, number of metastatic sites, and clinical response to treatment. In patients with a low serum CEA and a low value for this biomarker index, both of these values increased immediately after the chemotherapy treatment, an apparent discordance when there was otherwise evidence of tumor response. Such initial increase of serum tumor markers as a result of chemotherapy should not be considered as a failure.

Tumor-Specific Markers

There have been many attempts to isolate lung carcinoma-specific markers. In one of the earliest reports there was an antigen (X) that could be considered tumor-specific for lung cancer (Yachi et al., 1968), although related compounds were present in other carcinomas also. Specific antigens have also been suggested by delayed hypersensitivity studies (Hollinshead et al., 1975), heterologous antisera reactions (Watson et al., 1975; Ibrahim et al., 1980), and production of monoclonal antibodies by fusion of patients' lymphocytes from hilar and bronchial lymph nodes with rodent myeloma cells (Sikora and Wright, 1981).

Different lung carcinomas possess different specific antigens. However, using an undifferentiated lung tumor as antigen, Viza et al. (1975) demonstrated that heterologous antisera cross-reacted with all kinds of lung cancer. A highly specific marker for lung carcinomas (LuCa) was isolated from pleural effusions of a patient with squamous cell carcinoma. Its active component was of molecular weight 43,000–68,000 (Micksche et al., 1982). LuCa was present in sera at the following frequencies for patients with different lung carcinomas: 100% for squamous cell, 73% for adenocarcinoma and 67% for small-cell carcinomas. Serum levels of LuCa correlated with the clinical course of the disease.

Non-Small-Cell Carcinomas

Several monoclonal antibodies raised to non-small-cell carcinomas of the lung reacted with non-small-cell and other carcinomas, but not with normal tissues tested by Fickert et al. (1983). One of these antibodies (mab S-7) was related to glycoproteins of molecular weight of 48,000 and 180,000. Two other monoclonal antibodies produced against a human large-cell carcinoma cell line reacted with 11 of 13 non-small-cell carcinomas, but with none of 11 small-cell carcinomas tested (Mulshine et al., 1983). They reacted also with 7 of 8 melanomas, an osteogenic sarcoma, and a renal cell sarcoma, but not with other human neoplasms or normal adult tissues tested immunohistochemically.

Another monoclonal antibody (Ks1/9) raised against human adenocarcinoma cell line P3x63Ag8 reacted specifically with adenocarcinoma of lung and not with other malignant tumors or normal tissues (Varki et al., 1984).

Squamous cell carcinoma antigens

Squamous cell carcinoma is the most frequent lung tumor. A specific antiserum to squamous cell carcinoma was produced in rabbits (Kelly and Levy, 1980) and by hybridomas (Jothy et al., 1982). A monoclonal antibody was selectively specific only for bronchogenic squamous cell carcinomas (Brenner et al., 1982). In a group of glycoproteins studied by Wolf et al. (1981) there was one distinct antigen for squamous cel carcinomas. These lung carcinoma-associated glycoproteins had units with a molecular weight of approximately 43,000.

Adenocarcinoma markers

A glycoprotein specific for adenocarcinoma of the lung was isolated from a crude cell-free tumor extract by Gaffar et al. (1979). It had a molecular weight of 76,000 and consisted of three subunits, each with a molecular weight of 25,000.

Manganese-containinng superoxide dismutase activity can be considered as a marker for pulmonary adenocarcinomas. It has been found to be significantly higher in adenocarcinoma than in uninvolved lung tissues (Iizuka et al., 1984).

Alveolar cell carcinoma antigens

An alveolar cell carcinoma antigen, studied with sheep antiserum to a particle pallet from the tumor, cross-reacted with antigens in the sera of patients with lung carcinomas and of some patients with Hodgkin's lymphoma. Using the immunodiffusion method, Mohr et al. (1974) detected alveolar cell carcinoma antibodies in 11 of 13 patients with this tumor and in 3 of 5 patients with adenocarcinoma. This antigen was also demonstrated on lymphocytes of patients with alveolar cell carcinoma who had extensive involvement by tumor or widespread metastases (Mohr et al., 1975).

Small-Cell Carcinomas

CEA

Goslin et al. (1983) reported that in patients with small-cell carcinomas tissue CEA correlated with CEA in the serum; serum CEA was elevated in 86% of 21 patients with evidence of CEA in tumor tissues. In 27 cases without tissue CEA, only 3 patients had elevated serum CEA. There was more extensive disease and higher incidence of metastases when CEA was demonstrated in the tissues.

Neuron-specific enolase (NSE)

Neuron-specific enolase is a marker for neuroendocrine tumors. It was demonstrated immunohistochemically in the cells of 2 of 3 small-cell carcinomas examined by Wick et al. (1983).

In the serum of healthy individuals NSE ranged from 1.3 to 3.0 ng/ml in a study by Ariyoshi et al. (1983a), with a mean of 2.1 ± 0.4 ng/ml. Positive serum NSE levels (exceeding 7.5 ng/ml concentration) were observed in 90% of 10 oat cell carcinoma patients and in 40% of 10 patients with the intermediate cell carcinoma subtype. In addition, in 54 non-small-cell carcinoma patients examined only 11% had positive serum NSE. Such elevated levels of NSE occurred in the serum of the patients with carcinomas at an advanced clinical stage. As a marker NSE levels in serum corresponded to the clinical course during treatment. The neuroendocrine type of these tumors has been demonstrated immunohistochemically (Sheppard et al., 1984), and NSE thus served as a marker for undifferentiated small-cell tumors.

Physalaemin

Physalaemin is an amphibian tachykinin. A similar peptide was found in a human small-cell carcinoma by Lazarus et al. (1983). The tumor physalaemin was immunologically and functionally similar to the amphibian one. They both induced contractions of isolated guinea pig ileum. This may be potential tumor marker for small-cell carcinomas of the lung and perhaps for other tumors with neuroendocrine activity.

Bombesin

Bombesin, a neuropeptide in brain, has also been detected in all 17 cell lines from small-cell carcinomas examined by Moody et al. (1981). It ranged from 0.02 to 12.7 pmoles/mg of soluble protein in small-cell carcinomas, but less than 0.01 in adenocarcimas and large-cell and squamous cell carcinomas and mesotheliomas. Elevated blood levels corresponded with the extent of tumor burden.

Bombesin is present in the endocrine cells of fetal and neonatal lung, but is present in decreased amounts in the adult tissues or is absent. Thus, it is an oncofetal tumor marker. It is of interest that bombesin activity as a potent mitogen for Swiss 3T3 cells is related to the mitogenic effect of the chemically diverse tumor promoters phorbol esters and teleocidin, thus indicating some role for this hormone in carcinogenesis (Rozengurt and Collins, 1983). Bombesin may have an effect on malignant neoplasms that is similar to that of other growth factors. It may promote or sustain the tumor by "autocrine circuit" (Rozengurt and Collins, 1983), where the same cell that produces bombesin becomes influenced by it.

Modified ribonucleosides

One or more nucleosides were elevated in the urine of 96% of 28 patients with small-cell carcinomas examined by Waalkes et al. (1982). Two or less were elevated in 91% of 11 patients with limited disease. In 94% of 17 patients with extensive disease three or more nucleosides were elevated. The survival time correlated with the frequency of urinary nucleosides. The patients survived 24 months with two or less but only 10 months with three or more elevated nucleosides. A composite score derived from the nucleoside values reflected tumor burden and clinical response to therapy. This approach provided less variable results than CEA determinations.

Oat-cell carcinoma antigens

Specificity of membrane antigens was established with a rabbit antiserum to a purified fraction of oat cell carcinoma plasma membranes by Bell and Seetharam (1976). This antigen was not present in other kinds of lung tumors, but it was detected in all seven oat cell carcinomas examined. Some of these antigens extracted by Harlozinska et al. (1980) with perchloride acid were not related to CEA.

Oncogenes

Oncogene c-K-ras 2

It is not yet established that the oncogene mutation is more than a phenomenon that has occurred in a few lung carcinoma cell lines (Nakano et al., 1984). If it were a more general event the altered c-K-*ras*2 gene with the point mutations and the expression of an altered protein p21 with the substitutions of single amino acids at positions 12 and 61 would represent a true tumor-specific marker. A specifity of some sort is apparent where in the same patient *K-ras* is activated in the tumor cells but not in the normal cells (Santos et al., 1984).

c-myc

There was c-*myc* gene amplification in 8 of 18 lung carcinoma cell lines examined by Little et al. (1983). Among those 8 cell lines 5 were derived from small-cell carcinomas. As a marker the product of c-*myc* amplification would be characteristic with its excess, not specific for malignant neoplasms, since c-H-*ras* and c-K-*ras* amplification has been observed in normal animals (Chattopadhyay et al., 1982).

ORAL TUMORS

Oral Squamous Cell Carcinomas

Serum thymidine kinase activity was elevated in patients with oral squamous cell carcinomas studied by Scully (1982). The serum levels were higher if the regional lymph nodes were also involved. The enzyme activity decreased postoperatively in patients without recurrent tumor.

Genus-specific antigens of human papillomavirus were demonstrated immunohistochemically by Jenson et al. (1982a) in 18 of 29 verrucal papillomas, 2 of 2 multiple papillomas, and 3 of 5 condylomata but not in keratoacanthomas. The role of the virus in oral squamous cell carcinogenesis is not known. There is evidence of the presence of two different herpes simplex virus type 1 late antigens (Shillitoe et al. 1984). One reacted with an IgA, the other with IgM antibodies.

Salivary Gland Tumors

Seifert and Caselitz (1983) demonstrated histochemically the presence of CEA in 10 of 16 adenocarcinomas, in 3 of 4 adenoid cystic carcinomas, in 5 of 7 mucoepidermoid tumors, in 6 of 10 squamous cell carcinomas, and in 9 of 21 pleomorphic adenomas. TPA was present in the ducts of normal salivary glands and in the epidermoid part of the mucoepidermoid tumors. It is possible that elevated levels of these markers are present in the serum also.

Using immunohistochemical and immunodiffusion methods Nakazato et al. (1982) demonstrated that pleomorphic adenomas of the salivary glands contain "nervous system-specific protein" S-100, the glial fibrillary acidic protein (GFAP), and astroprotein. Normal salivary glands did not contain these markers. The GFAP has some heterogeneity when tested by immunodiffusion. Thus a variant of GFAP may be related to pleomorphic adenomas of the salivary glands.

TUMORS OF THE NASOPHARYNX AND PARANASAL SINUSES

Nasopharyngeal Carcinomas

These tumors represent a rather homogeneous group. They all produce keratin (Gusterson et al., 1983), in spite of their degree of differentiation. Undifferentiated nasopharyngeal carcinomas can thus be differentiated from lymphomas, which do not produce histochemically demonstrable keratin.

MS-Ag, a Membrane Antigen

A membrane-soluble antigen (MS-Ag) was isolated from cultured nasopharyngeal carcinoma cells by Tsukuda et al. (1980). Cellular immune responses of nonimmunized and immunized mice indicated the specificity of this antigen.

Proteins

Two unique proteins with a molecular weight of approximately 40,000 were found in sera (80%) of patients with this tumor and in sera (80%) of patients with Burkitt's lymphoma (Gazitt et al., 1981).

Virus-like Components

Cells of nasopharyngeal carcinomas studied by Kufe et al. (1973c) contained RNA sequences homologous to Rauscher leukemia virus. Such RNA sequences were present also in the cells of Burkitt's lymphoma. There is some evidence that an RNA also occurs in the tumor cells (Arnold et al., 1981). Since there was a correlation between RNA coronavirus and the presence of Epstein-Barr virus (EBV) nuclear antigen in these tumors, there may be some interaction of these viruses in the pathogenesis of the nasopharyngeal carcinomas.

EBV antibodies against viral capsid and early antigen were increased in 85% of the patients studied by Neel et al. (1983) who had tumors of types 2 and 3 according to WHO classification. Such increased serum titers of the antibodies were observed in only 16% of patients with type 1 tumors. Follow-up with evaluation of antibody titers can detect recurrence of the tumor after therapy. It may be appropriate to suspect occult primary tumor with an elevated serum titer of EBV antibodies.

In testing IgA and IgG antibodies to EBV capsid (VCA) and early antigen (EA), there was revealed a stepwise rise of all antibodies with progression of the disease (Ho et al., 1982). The relative sensitivities of detection of EBV antigens by these antibodies was as follows: IgA to VCA 95% and IgA to EA 78%, followed by sensitivity IgG to EA, and the least discriminating, IgG sensitivity to VCA.

Papilloma Virus Antigens in Paranasal Sinus Carcinomas

Human papilloma virus (HPV) antigens were detected by Syrjanen et al. (1983b) in cells of paranasal sinus carcinomas. Since nasal squamous cell papillomas can transform to carcinomas, it is possible that HPV plays a role in the pathogenesis of this tumor. Marker antibodies to HPV are available for further study of the relationship between HPV and tumors of paranasal sinuses.

GASTROINTESTINAL TUMORS

Besides AFP and CEA there are numerous other markers related to malignant neoplasms of the gastrointestinal system (Klavins, 1983). Most of these markers have been studied in patients with colon carcinoma and related to CEA or in patients with hepatoma and related to AFP.

Carcinomas of the Stomach

Oncofetal Markers

An antiserum to second-trimester human fetal tissues was used for the determination of the sequence of expression of oncofetal antigens in the development of gastric mucosal dysplasia (Higgins et al., 1983a). Antiserum from a rabbit was absorbed with normal adult tissue extracts and HT-29 colon carcinoma cells to remove the activity of certain antigenic determinants shared by adult stomach and second-trimester fetal colon. After the absorption this antiserum reacted with 33% of atrophic gastritis cells, 38% of intestinal metaplasia cells, and 82% of cells of gastric epithelial dysplasia. The antiserum did not react with normal gastric mucosal cells. The nature of the antigen is not known.

CEA

Elevated serum CEA levels occurred in 32% of patients with gastric carcinomas studied by Kjaer and Fischerman (1976). Elevated serum levels of the common oncofetal markers HCG (Braunstein et al., 1973) and AFP (McIntire et al., 1975) occurred in 24% and 15% of the gastric carcinoma patients, respectively.

Preoperative serum CEA concentration was a significant prognostic parameter for postoperative survival of 390 patients studied by Staab et al. (1982). High CEA values were associated with poor prognosis. Other statistically significant parameters were age of the patient, tumor extension, and stages of disease (I–IV, UICC). CEA determinations in the gastric juice were of little value as a diagnostic aid but contributed to identification of patients at risk (Nitti et al., 1983). In 88% of 8 carcinoma patients gastric juice had CEA levels greater than 100 ng/ml. In all 5 patients with epithelial dysplasia and in all 6 with intestinal metaplasia CEA values in gastric juice were above 100 ng/ml).

The presence of CEA was demonstrated in 92% of 119 primary carcinomas examined by Hockey et al. (1984). This again indicates a high frequency of CEA production by gastric carcinomas, although serum CEA was elevated in only 32% of patients with this tumor (Kjaer and Fischerman, 1976). Of the 119 patients with primary gastric carcinomas, 81 had metastases and of these 83% contained CEA in metastatic tumors. In two cases tumor cells were identified by the presence of CEA in lymph nodes, which before this study were considered free of metastases. CEA was not expressed by all metastatic tumors, indicating phenotypic diversity of the tumor cell clones.

TPA

Elevated serum TPA was present in 77% of 39 patients with gastric carcinoma (Wagner et al., 1982). Serum CEA was elevated in 46% of 35 patients in this study. In a control group of 52 surgical patients false positive rate for CEA was 23% and for TPA 15%.

Fetal sulfoglycoprotein

This tumor marker (FSA) is significant in detection of stomach carcinomas (Häkkinen et al., 1980). In a mass screening of 53,020 people, 47 malignant gastric neoplasms were detected, 15 in the early stages. These early carcinomas could not be detected by conventional clinical means. Thus, prognosis with early detection and immediate treatment of these patients is greatly improved.

FSA is immunologically related to, but not identical to, CEA (Häkkinen (1972). This marker was present in the superficial epithelial cells of fetal intestinal tract and occasionally in normal adult epithelial cells or cells associated with gastric ulcer. It is present regularly in the gastric carcinoma cell secretions.

Tumor-Associated Markers

Using a panel of tumor markers—CEA, pseudouridine phosphohexose isomerase, C-reactive protein, alpha 1-A glycoprotein, and gamma-glutamyl transpeptidase—89% of 76 gastric carcinoma patients were detected at a marker score level of 10% false-positives among the controls by De Mello et al. (1982).

SGA

A sulfated glycoprotein (SGA) was detected in stomach carcinomas, in cells of intestinal metaplasia of stomach mucosa, and in some intestinal epithelial cells (Bara et al., 1978). This marker was not present in poorly differentiated gastric tumors. The relationship of this protein to fetal sulfoglycoprotein (Häkkinen, 1972) is not known.

Serum DNA-binding protein (64DP)

This universal tumor-associated marker (Mitomi et al., 1982) was studied in 26 patients with gastric carcinoma in different stages. There was no correlation between serum 64DP levels and the stages. In 29 patients studied by serial 64DP determinations, the serum levels decreased approximately 3 weeks after surgical treatment but did not return to normal levels.

Serum Ferritin

Serum ferritin was found to be elevated in 44% of patients with recurrent gastric carcinoma (Tomoda et al., 1982). It was measured using antihuman placental ferritin antiserum.

Tumor-Specific Markers

A unique antigen was not present in the tumors but was detected in gastric secretions of stomach cancer patients studied by Deutsch et al. (1973). It differed from CEA.

The sera of gastric cancer patients contained an antigen with 3-oxyanthranilic acid in a study by Korosteleva et al. (1976). This marker was not present in sera of normal individuals. It appeared in the patients' serum early in the disease.

A specific protein was isolated using rabbit antiserum to aqueous extract of stomach cancer (Furukawa et al., 1977). This was not a glycoprotein and did not cross-react with CEA. This antigen was present also in the urine of patients with gastric cancer.

Carcinomas of the Small Intestine

AFP may be tested for carcinomas of the small intestine. In the serum of a patient with an adenocarcinoma of the ileum and coexistent Crohn disease, AFP rose from 8,612 kU/liter to 15,540 kU/liter (normal considered as less than 10 kU/liter). This increased serum AFP level was associated with an increase in CEA to 963 ng/ml (Leader and Jass, 1984). In this case the liver was involved by extensive metastases. Therefore, it is possible that the source of AFP could have been the liver and not necessarily the tumor cells. Since CEA was elevated in the serum, it too can be considered a potential marker for carcinomas of the small intestine.

Colon Cancer

Oncofetal Markers

CEA

CEA is the best-known marker for colon carcinomas and has been effectively applied in follow-up of patients (Go and Zamcheck, 1982). Serum HCG is also elevated in 16% of patients with colorectal carcinoma (Cabnal et al., 1981), while AFP is elevated in only 5% of the cases studied (Waldmann and McIntire, 1974).

Preoperative serum CEA levels correlated with Dukes classification in 124 patients examined (Midiri et al., 1983). The mean CEA values for stages A, B, C, and D were 7.8, 30.3, 58.1, and 134.3 ng/ml, respectively. There was no correlation of serum CEA levels with histologic grading.

Although CEA is a marker for recurrence about 6 months before other clinical manifestations appear, the question remains about the usefulness of the postoperative screening of patients (Carlsson et al., 1983). Most of such recurrences may not be curable. In some cases decreasing serum CEA during chemotherapy does not reflect complete remission, and increasing concentration does not always indicate recurrence (Persijn, 1982). It may be more promising to use Goldenberg's radioimmunodetection method to select patients for surgical treatment after primary resection (Begent et al., 1983). It may be possible to localize the recurrent tumor before it becomes evident clinically.

^{131}I-labeled heteroantibodies to CEA localized in the sites of colon carcinoma, and thus these lesions were detected (Goldenberg et al., 1983a). By application of total-body photoscans, primary colorectal carcinoma was localized in 83% of 12 cases, and 90% of 53 metastatic sites were detected. The false-positive rate was less than 4% and false-negative rates ranged between 9% and 14%. Radioimmunodetection contributed significantly to the clinical staging and evaluation of therapeutic response and recurrence, confirmed the findings of less specific tumor detection methods, and indicated the sites of the recurrence when the serum CEA was rising. The latter approach may justify a second-look operation in appropriate cases. There has been some benefit from second-look surgery (Steele et al., 1980). After two successive increases in serum CEA in 18 patients, 15 were explored surgically. Of the 15, 4 were treated in an attempt to cure and 2 of these were free of disease 13 and 24 months later. The cure rate was 13% of 15 patients treated by second-look surgery.

In an attempt to apply CEA determinations to prognosis (Steele et al., 1982), it was found that there was a greater probability of recurrence if the preoperative serum CEA of colon carcinoma patients was greater than 5 ng/ml. Such CEA determinations were not prognostically significant for the patients with rectal carcinomas. A rising trend of elevated serum CEA was more frequently associated with a recurrence. However, in patients selected for a curative resection of the tumor there was no correlation between the subsequent survival and the preoperative CEA levels (Lewi et al., 1984).

CEA doubling times were calculated to assess the effect of therapy and survival by Staab et al. (1982b). Analysis was done of patients with recurrent carcinoma. In 76% of 114 cases there was a linear relationship between time and log CEA increase. The doubling times were calculated within this log CEA period and the ranges were the following: 142–868 days with local recurrence or second primary, 47–231 days with visceral metastases except liver, 10–102 days with liver metastases, 54–60 days with bone metastases, and 598 days with brain metastases. While mean survival time was 7.0 ± 9.4 CEA doubling times, for patients with liver metastases it was significantly longer—17.4 ± 9.4 CEA doubling times.

Another approach to calculating the limits of CEA for the estimation of tumor response to therapy is to use the following formula (Lokich et al., 1984): square root of 2 × the variability about the mean yields CEA variability relative to the baseline CEA level.

Monthly serum CEA determinations in follow-up have been recommended for the first 2 years and every 3 months for the next 3 years (Minton, 1982). After 5 years, annual serum CEA determinations and colonoscopy or barium enema have been recommended. It is estimated that 2 or 3 recurrences appear during the first 2 years and 9 of 10 before 5 years.

Complimentary to CEA is Tennessee antigen (Brockamp et al., 1982). It was elevated in serum at a rate of 91% when serum levels of 23 patients with rectal carcinomas were normal. On the other hand CEA levels were elevated in 2 of 6 patients with normal Tennessee antigen concentration.

TPA

Serum TPA was elevated in 62% of 60 colorectal carcinoma patients studied by Wagner et al. (1982). In this same group, serum CEA was elevated at a rate of 64%. In a control group of 52 surgical patients false TPA values occurred at a rate of 15% and false-positive CEA values at a rate of 23%.

FG 3 antigen

Antiserum to this Fucα1→3Gal linkage reacted with several kinds of normal mouse tissues and 71% of 17 human colonic adenocarcinomas. It did not react with any other colon epithelial cells but did react with 3 teratocarcinoma stem cell lines, indicating its embryonic nature (Miyauchi et al., 1982).

Oncofetal markers limited to colonic carcinomas

Using rabbit antiserum to tissues of second trimester human fetus, an antigen was detected, cross-reacting with adenomas and carcinomas of colon (Higgins et al., 1981). This antigen was not AFP or CEA. It increased in frequency in adenomas as they progressed toward carcinomas.

An antiserum prepared against fetal tissues (Higgins et al., 1983a) reacted with a distinctly different frequency when exposed to various types of colonic adenomas (Higgins et al., 1983b). The antigen(s) appeared to increase in frequency when the adenomas progressed to more atypical types. The antigen-positive cells increased from 18% to 43% to 70% in cell cultures from tubular, villotubular, and villous adenomas, respectively.

Other oncofetal markers in the colon that are distinct from AFP and CEA are an antigen (CSAp) obtained from a human colonic carcinoma xenograft

(Pant et al., 1977) and a nonsulfated mucin with a molecular weight of 70,000–100,000 (Ma et al., 1980).

Using a monoclonal antibody, a monosialoganglioside was detected in colon carcinoma by Magnani et al. (1982). This ganglioside contained sialylated lacto-N-fucopentose II. It was detected in 57% of 21 adenocarcinomas of the colon, 4 of 5 gastric carcinomas, and 4 of 7 pancreatic carcinomas. This marker was present in human meconium and thus may be of embryonic origin. Other monoclonal antibodies produced to a colorectal adenocarcinoma, or to cell membranes of a metastatic colon adenocarcinoma, also reacted with a monosialoganglioside fraction in 60–90% of the colorectal and pancreatic carcinomas examined (Lindholm et al., 1983). This antigen was not detected in normal colonic mucosa or other tissues tested.

There is also an oncofetal thymidine kinase, detected by Balis et al. (1981). This phase-specific isoenzyme was present in human placenta, in colon carcinoma cells, and in fibroblasts of patients with hereditary familial polyposis.

In human red blood and colon carcinoma cells there have been found glycolipids that constitute an embryonal antigen (SSEA-1). This antigen fraction in carcinoma contained a novel polyfucosyl structure (Hakomori et al., 1981). A monoclonal antibody to it could recognize this antigen in all human colon carcinoma tissues examined immunohistochemically (Shi et al., 1984). SSEA-1 was present in the lower crypts of normal colonic mucosa, but in the adjacent areas of the tumor SSEA-1 was also present in the surface epithelium and upper crypts.

Tumor-Associated Markers

Monoclonal antibodies are produced against colon carcinomas as they are against various other malignant neoplasms. Some of these antibodies may be specific against the corresponding malignant neoplasm. A hybridoma antibody against a colorectal carcinoma cell line was inhibited more than 19% from binding to its antigen by sera from 33 patients with advanced colorectal carcinomas at a frequency of 72%. The average inhibition of binding by individuals including heavy smokers, without evidence of disease was below 10%. Two pancreatic carcinoma patients had serum with inhibition greater than 19% and the sera of 2 gastric cancer patients inhibited binding at a rate of 10–19% (Koprowski et al., 1981). These studies indicate that in the serum of colon carcinoma patients there is a specific antigen, a potential specific marker. In subsequent studies (Sears et al., 1982) it was determined that monoclonal antibody can detect a tumor-associated antigen in 70% of patients with advanced colorectal carcinoma.

Another cytotoxic monoclonal antibody (CCOL1) reacted with cytotoxicity to only one other colon carcinoma cell line besides the inducer indicating its individuality (Kaszurbowski et al., 1984). The antigen, a glycoprotein, was present in other colon cancer tissues and in smaller amounts in normal epithelial cells.

Lactosylsphingosine

Increased titers of antibodies to lactosylsphingosine were present in all 39 patients with colorectal carcinoma studied by Jozwiak and Koscielak (1982). The antibody titers decreased in 32% of patients between 3 and 6 months postoperatively, and 85% of 13 such patients were free of the disease up to 2 years. If the high level of antibodies persisted longer than 6 months, there were recurrences. In 40% of the cases high titers of antibodies to lactosylsphingosine preceded the increase of serum CEA.

Zinc glycinate marker (ZGM)

ZGM has been isolated from a colon carcinoma. It differed from AFP and CEA and had a molecular weight greater than 2,000,000 and α_2 electrophoretic mobility (Saravis et al., 1978). It was present in adenocarcinomas of the gastrointestinal tract. Using immunofluorescence microscropy, ZGM was also demonstrated in the deep crypts of the villi of grossly nonmalignant tissues.

Acute phase reactant proteins

Serum protein hexose, ceruloplasmin, transferrin, α-1 antitrypsin, seromucoid, and haptoglobin reflected the disease status of patients with colorectal carcinoma studied by Walker and Gray (1983). Of these proteins, serum protein hexose had the greatest value as a tumor marker. Combined with CEA determinations, it revealed the greatest number of patients with colorectal carcinoma. In spite of detection of recurrence earlier than with other means, the benefit was limited to a few patients (Gray and Walker, 1983). There was a low incidence of successful removal of the tumor at the second operation.

A 220,000- to 240,000-dalton glycoprotein that reacted with a monoclonal antibody B72.3 was reported by Stramignoni et al. (1983). This antibody was raised against membrane-enriched extracts of human breast carcinomas, and it reacted with 82% of 17 colon carcinomas, but only a few percent of the cells of 18 adenomas examined reacted with it. When the antibody was diluted, 50% of 16 carcinomas reacted with it and none of the 46 adenomas. This antibody may be useful in certain cases for differentiating adenomas from carcinomas.

When haptoglobin 2-1 alone was compared with CEA by multivariate analysis, the correlation between elevated haptoglobin and colorectal cancer was higher than that between CEA and colorectal carcinomas (Cherubini et al., 1982). Elevated serum heptoglobin was found in some early stages of carcinoma when CEA was not increased.

The frequency of detecting colon carcinomas has been increased by using a panel of different markers (De Mello et al., 1982). When serum was assayed for elevated levels of CEA, pseudouridine phosphohexose isomerase, C-reactive protein, α-1-A glycoprotein, and γ-glutamyl transpeptidase, 90% of 99 patients with colorectal carcinoma were detected at a level of marker scores such that in the controls the false-positive rate was 10%.

By combining leukocyte adherence inhibition with CEA determination, sensitivity was increased to 91% with a 68% specificity (Payne et al., 1983).

Colon-specific antigen-p (CSAp)

There was an increased sensitivity for the presence of a tumor marker when CEA determination was combined with the determination of serum CSAp by Pant et al. (1982). Both CEA and CSAp are found to occur at elevated serum levels in patients with malignant neoplasms other than colorectal cancer. Since CSAp is elevated more frequently in carcinomas of the colon than in other malignant neoplasms, it can serve well to supplement CEA monitoring of patients with colorectal cancer. Assuming CEA cutoff at 5 ng/ml, CSAp was present in 14% of CEA-negative cases. On the other hand, CSAp was not elevated in 25% of colonic adenoma cases positive for CEA.

UDP-galactosyltransferase (GT)

Serum GT was found to increase more frequently than CEA in patients with colon carcinoma (Munjal et al., 1981).

Deoxythymidine-5'-triphosphatase (dTTP)

The enzyme activity of dTTP in the serum of colon cancer patients has been found to correlate with the clinical course of the disease and tumor burden (Dahlmann and Pompecki, 1984). The highest dTTP activity levels were in patients with Duke's stage B and C tumors. This marker in combination with CEA increased the percentage of patients who could be followed up with one of them.

Ornithine decarboxylase

It is possible to identify family members who carry the genotype for familial clonic polyposis, (Luk and Baylin, 1984). Colonic mucosal biopsies of carriers contained significantly higher amounts of ornithine decarboxylase activity than did those of normal controls. The distinction was striking. The patients had more activities > 2.5 nM/mg/hr and the controls less than that amount. The enzyme activity was higher in cases of dysplastic polyps than in those without dysplasia. The increase in ornithine decarboxylase activity was related to the hyperproliferation of mucosal epithelial cells in familial colonic polyposis.

CA 19-9

This universal tumor-associated marker was compared with CEA (Kuusela et al., 1984). There was no correlation between these markers for colorectal carcinomas. The sensitivity of CA 19-9 was 36%. The specificity at these levels for CA 19-9 was 97% and for CEA 70%. Thus for follow-up CEA may be preferred to CA 19-9. However, in cases where CEA production is nonspecific, CA 19-9 would serve well as a marker for follow-up of patients with colorectal cancer. This marker may be especially useful for patients with advancing colorectal carcinoma (Ritts et al., 1984). CA 19-9 is found to be elevated in the serum of patients with advanced adenocarcinoma of the upper gastrointestinal tract, as well as pancreatic and liver carcinomas.

Tumor-Specific Markers

Tumor-specific antigens have been demonstrated with immunoelectrophoretic studies of gastric and colon carcinomas (Harlozinska et al., 1975). These antigens were not present in fetal gastrointestinal tissues. It has been suggested (Miller and Tom, 1980) that colon carcinoma-specific antigens are present among those solubilized by 3 M KC1. A unique polyfucosyl structure was detected in a colon adenocarcinoma by Hakomori et al. (1981).

Sera of colon carcinoma patients have been found to contain antibodies to a glycoprotein (GP40) that can be isolated from the serum immune complexes of patients with Burkitt's lymphoma (Gazitt et al., 1983). These antibodies correlated with the extent of the disease, decreasing as the carcinoma progressed and increasing in remission as a result of therapy.

Four monoclonal antibodies raised against human colonic carcinoma cells have reacted exclusively with adenocarcinomas of the colon (Sakamoto et al., 1983). This indicates the presence in these tumors of possible specific antigens.

When human monoclonal antibodies were used 8 specific antisera reacted only with tumor tissues (McCabe et al., 1984). Such human monoclonal antisera as distinct from murine antisera, may be applicable as markers and may be more readily applicable in new immunological therapeutic modalities.

It is possible that adenocarcinoma-specific substances are in the monosialogangliosides. Monoclonal antibodies to an adenocarcinoma cell line have reacted selectively with colorectal adenocarcinoma cells (Lindholm et al., 1983). The antigens corresponding to some of these monoclonal antibodies were in the monosialoganglioside fraction of the tumors.

Altered colonic mucoproteins

A colonic mucoprotein (CMA) isolated from colon carcinoma has been found to differ from normal CMA. The CMA from carcinoma tissues had a 40% higher content of aspartic acid and 40% lower threonine content than normal CMA. There were significant differences in the content of other amino acids also. It was suggested that CMA in colonic carcinoma is a neoantigen, expressed by a new or altered sequence of DNA (Gold, 1977).

Similarly, from lectin-binding studies it was concluded that there was a unique mucin in colon carcinoma cells (Boland et al., 1982). It was detected by binding with peanut agglutinin Arachis hypogaea, a lectin with high affinity for a carbohydrate structure normally not exposed in tissues. This lectin did not bind to the goblet cell mucin of normal colonic epithelium but had an affinity for the epithelial cells adjacent to the carcinoma.

Basic antigen (pI 7.8)

This is a colon carcinoma antigen detected in cytosol and nuclear fractions (Taylor et al., 1980). It was not related to CEA or normal human tissues.

β_2-Microglobulin-associated antigen

This antigen was isolated from colon carcinoma. Except for specificity, it had characteristics similar to those of β_2-microglobulin-associated specific antigens in breast carcinoma, melanoma, and hepatoma (Thomson et al., 1978). This appareent neoantigen was not related to CEA (Thomson et al., 1980).

A specific adenosine deaminase

Colon carcinomas have been found to produce an isoenzyme that differs by its molecular weight from the enzyme in normal colonic mucosa. It was different from the normal mucosal enzyme in the extent of neutralization by an immune serum raised against normal enzyme (Balis et al., 1981).

γ-Glutamyltransferases

An enzyme with reduced affinity to concanavalin A (Con A) and asialo isomer without affinity to Con A have been found in colonic adenocarcinomas (Huseby and Eide, 1983). These forms did not differ in size or antigenicity from the enzyme in normal tissues. Evidently they have an altered carbohydrate component.

Chromosome abnormalities

Chromosome abnormalities have been detected with structural and numerical changes of chromosomes 7 and 12 of colonic adenocarcinoma cells (Ochi et al., 1983). Since proto-oncogene is located on chromosome 12, changes of this chromosome may in some way induce the expression of this oncogene. Chromosome 7 abnormalities are found in other tumors also.

Oncogenes

An alteration of the c-K-*ras*2 gene in some human colon and lung carcinoma cell lines has been reported (Der and Cooper, 1983). Activation of the c-K-*ras*2 gene was associated with two different point mutations (Capon et al., 1983). Thus a single amino acid substitution at positions 12 and 61 of the p21 would provide a unique tumor-specific marker. The extent of this alteration in colon carcinoma is not known. In 29 primary carcinomas of colon, lung, and urinary bladder there was no evidence of gene mutations producing amino acid substitution in p21 at position 12 (Feinberg et al., 1983).

Chromosomes of malignant neuroendocrine cells from a human colon carcinoma contained amplified copies of c-*myc* (Alitalo et al., 1983).

CARCINOMAS OF THE PANCREAS

Oncofetal Markers

Elevated levels of AFP (Waldmann and McIntire, 1974), CEA (Ona et al., 1973), and HCG (Braunstein et al., 1973) occur in the sera of patients with pancreatic carcinoma at frequencies of 23%, 85%, and 50%, respectively. Serum CEA was markedly elevated (6400 ng/ml) in a patient with a signet ring carcinoma (Tracey et al., 1984). This is a rare tumor of the pancreas.

α-HCG-reactive antigens were detected in 75% of 56 functioning malignant endocrine tumors (Heitz et al., 1983). They were observed with the immunohistochemical method in only 1 of 67 functioning benign tumors. There was no evidence of β-HCG.

The diagnostic rate of pancreatic carcinoma was increased to 100% by combined cytologic examination and CEA determination in specimens obtained by percutaneous fine-needle aspiration biopsy (Tatsuta et al., 1983).

Acinar cells probably contribute to the elevated serum CEA. The highest values (2,500–6,100 ng/ml) were found in two patients with acinar cell carcinomas (Horie et al., 1984).

In both serological and immunhistochemical studies of CEA in pancreatic carcinoma, as well as in other tumors, it is important to consider the possibility of an interference with a nonspecific cross-reacting antigen (NCA). While NCA was present in normal pancreatic ducts, CEA was not demonstrated using monoclonal antibodies to it (Tsutsumi et al., 1984).

Duct Cell Carcinoma-Associated Antigen

A monoclonal antibody to human pancreatic duct cells (HP-DU-1) were found to react with antigens of normal ducts, all adenocarcinomas, and fetal pancreatic duct cells of 12 weeks gestation (Parsa et al., 1982). This antibody reacted with a cell surface antigen and may represent a potential marker for pancreatic duct cell carcinomas.

T Antigen

This marker, precursor of the MN blood group antigens, can be used in the differential diagnosis of pancreatic carcinoma and acute pancreatitis (Springer, 1984). Of 26 patients with pancreatic carcinoma, 88% had a positive delayed hypersensitivity reaction to T antigen. None of the 13 patients with acute pancreatitis had a positive reaction to this antigen.

Pancreatic Oncofetal Antigen (POA)

With the use of two-dimensional immunoelectrophoresis, an antigen (POA) has been demonstrated only in fetal pancreas and in sera of patients with pancreatic carcinoma or in extracts of pancreatic tumor tissues (Banwo et al., 1974). It had an α_2-electrophoretic mobility. In subsequent studies, its molecular weight was determined to be between 800,000 and 900,000 (Gelder et al., 1979) or 40,000 as determined by using polyacrylamide gel electrophoresis in the presence of sodium dodecyl sulfate (Hobbs et al., 1980). Although this tumor marker was also expressed by other neoplasms and was present in small amounts in sera of some healthy individuals, it was more useful than any other marker in diagnosis and follow-up of patients with pancreatic carcinoma (Hobbs et al., 1980).

An enzyme immunoassay was developed to study the POA in patients (Oguchi et al., 1984). With this method 72% of patients with pancreatic carcinoma were identified. POA above normal levels was present in sera of patients with other malignant neoplasms, but at a considerably lesser frequency.

There appear to be several POA species. The substances isolated by Gelder et al. (1979) and Oguchi et al. (1984) are probably the same. Their molecular weight is about 800,000 and they have other similar characteristics. POA reported by Hobbs et al. (1980) had a lower molecular weight and lacked a carbohydrate component.

A pancreatic carcinoma-associated antigen was isolated and purified from normal colonic mucosa (Shimano et al., 1983). It was identical immunologically to POA and had a molecular weight of approximately 600,000 daltons. This antigen was designated PCAAc. It was significantly elevated in the serum of patients with pancreatic carcinomas.

Pancreatic Carcinoma-Associated Antigen (PCAA)

PCAA is a glycoprotein with a molecular weight of 185,000 (Chu et al., 1977). PCAA was detected predominantly in the proliferative phase of the tumor cells, while CEA appeared diffusely distributed, predominantly in the cuboidal cells of the tumor, at the luminal border, and in mucin (Tan et al., 1981). It is not certain, but another known PCAA is probably different. It is a glycoprotein with a molecular weight of approximately 1,000,000, an isoelectric point of 4.7, and a sedimentation coefficient of 14S (Shimano et al., 1981). This PCAA was isolated from ascites fluid of a patient with pancreatic carcinoma. Serum levels of this marker were elevated in 67% of patients with carcinoma of the pancreas. With the use of immunoperoxidase microscopy with antiserum to PCAA, it was concluded that any metastatic tumor with a positive reaction is highly suggestive of pancreatic origin (Nadji et al., 1982).

Immunohistologically, PCAA is related to POA and is present also in the goblet cells of the intestinal tract (Maruyama et al., 1983).

Oncofetal Pancreatic Antigen (OPA)

Another oncofetal antigen with α_2-electrophoretic mobility (OPA) was isolated from the blood of patients with pancreatic carcinoma (Knapp, 1981). It is a protein with a molecular weight of 40,000 and is present in elevated amounts in the sera of patients with pancreatic carcinoma. OPA appeared useful in monitoring the disease.

The Oncofetal Antigen CAPI

We studied an antigen (CAPI) in an ammonium sulfate fraction (0-25%) from an aqueous extract of a pancreatic carcinoma (Mesa-Tejada et al., 1977). By immunoperoxidase microscopy CAPI was seen in all pancreatic carcinomas studied, in some other carcinomas, and in fetal colon. By the microcomplement fixation method a heterologous antiserum to CAPI cross-reacted with the sera of pancreatic carcinoma patients in a dilution of 1:16,000 (Klavins, 1981). At lower dilutions, this antiserum reacted with the sera of some normal individuals.

An Isoenzyme of Serum Ribonuclease With Acidic pI

This isoenzyme was detected in the serum of patients with pancreatic carcinoma or hepatoma, but not of patients with disease other than malignant tumors (Hishiki et al., 1984). It was present also in fetal pancrease and liver.

Tumor-Associated Markers

It has been found that there are pancreas carcinoma-associated antigens that can elicit antitumor immune reactions (Goldrosar et al., 1981), as demonstrated by the microplate leukocyte adherence inhibition assay.

An interspecies antigen was shared by pancreas carcinoma and normal pancreatic tissues of hamsters and human patients in a study by Sindelar et al. (1983). Xenoantiserum to normal hamster pancreas, appropriately absorbed with other tissues, reacted only with normal pancreas and pancreatic carcinomas.

DU-PAN-2

A pancreatic antigen, DU-PAN-2, defined by mice monoclonal antibodies, was detected in the serum of pancreatic cancer patients (Finn et al., 1984). It is a large mucin-like molecule.

CA19-9

This antigen is present at increased concentrations in the serum of patients with carcinomas. In the serum of 75% of pancreatic carcinoma patients CA19-9 was present in amounts above the normal range (Jalanko et al., 1984).

A Ribonuclease

Serum levels of a polycytidylic acid-specific ribonuclease were found significantly elevated in patients with pancreatic carcinoma (Warshaw et al., 1980). Thus, this enzyme can be used as another marker to follow the course of the disease. It may be applicable in differential diagnosis, since about 69% of patients with pancreatic cancer had an 800% elevation above normal. Serum enzyme values were also elevated in some patients with other malignant neoplasms (Reddi, 1980). However, in more recent studies (Weickmann et al., 1984) serum levels of the presumed pancreatic ribonuclease correlated better with kidney function than with the presence or absence of malignant neoplasms. Therefore, only in the absence of kidney disease, when no other marker is produced by a pancreatic carcinoma, may this enzyme be used to follow these patients.

Galactosyltransferase

Serum galactosyltransferase levels were found elevated in 67% of patients with carcinoma of the pancreas (Podolsky et al., 1981). When enzyme determination was combined with endoscopic retrograde cholangiopancrea tography, the sensitivity of the diagnosis approached 100%.

α-1-Antitrypsin

This serum protease inhibitor was elevated in 7 of 9 patients with pancreatic carcinomas studied by Tsuchiya et al. (1980). It was present in 36% of 33 tumor specimens from patients with islet cell carcinomas (Ordonez et al., 1983).

Ferritins

With the use of the anti-human placental ferritin in reversed passive hemagglutination method, serum ferritin levels were found to be elevated in 50% of patients with pancreatic carcinoma (Tomoda et al., 1982).

Tumor-Specific Markers

An antigen with a molecular weight of approximately 380,000 has been isolated from pancreatic carcinoma tissues (Kuntz and Archer, 1979). It was not detectable in normal pancreatic tissues and was not related to CEA. The presence of pancreatic carcinoma-specific antigen is suggested also by the special tumor immunity demonstrated using the leukocyte adherence inhibition assay (Tataryn et al., 1978) and murine monoclonal antibodies (Chin and Miller, 1984).

LIVER TUMORS

Of the two types of liver carcinomas, the hepatomas and the cholangiocarcinomas, the most frequently encountered is the hepatoma. In some cases the differentiation between pure hepatoma and pure cholangiocarcinoma is not possible.

Hepatomas

AFP

It has been estimated that about 80% of hepatoma patients have elevated serum AFP (Bloomer, 1980). The value of serial AFP determinations in patients at risk has been shown in the case of a symptomless patient with a continuous rise of AFP over a 3-month period (Heyward et al., 1983). All other liver tests for carcinoma were negative. At surgery a small tumor from the tip of the left lobe was removed. The patient was well at least 11 months postoperatively, and the AFP levels in the serum returned to normal.

In many cases of early hepatoma the serum AFP may be normal. Furthermore, a fall in serum AFP levels may be spontaneous, not associated with treatment in the early stages of this disease (Chen et al., 1984).

To differentiate between nonmalignant liver disease and hepatoma with border line elevated serum AFP, determination of AFP lectin-binding patterns is suggested (C.J. Smith et al., 1983). The glycosylation of AFP in nonmalignant liver diseases is similar to that in newborn liver, but differs in hepatomas.

Administration of pyridoxine and adenosine-5′-triphosphate (ATP) to alter the AFP production is another approach to differentiation of cirrhosis from early development of hepatoma (Watanabe and Nagashima, 1981). Serum AFP concentration decreased after simultaneous injection of pyridoxine and ATP in cirrhotic patients without hepatoma but did not decrease in hepatoma patients. A similar effect was observed in experimental animals.

Some AFP changes have been reflected to some degree in survival (Matsumoto et al., 1982). With serum AFP levels persistently below 200 ng/ml and well-differentiated hepatoma, the patients survived 34 months. With AFP increase to 1,000 ng/ml within 3–4 months the patients had moderately well differentiated tumors and survived about 16 months. If AFP increased to more than 10,000 ng/ml within a week, the patients had poorly differentiated hepatomas and survived only about 8 months.

CEA

CEA was elevated in the serum of 57% of 14 patients with hepatomas studied by Bell (1982). Since serum CEA and AFP are above normal levels in more than 50% of cases, it is suggested that for follow-up both markers be determined in cases where one is below the normal range. However, there is some doubt whether this CEA is the true oncofetal marker or cross-reactive differentiation antigen. Conventional rabbit anti-CEA antibodies would bind to the surface of bile canaliculi or normal hepatocytes (Hirohashi et al., 1983). Monoclonal antibodies to CEA did not bind to these cells.

Oncofetal Hepatoma Markers

With the use of an antiserum to human fetal liver cells, it was possible to demonstrate an oncofetal antigen in hepatomas (Weikang et al., 1977). This antigen was not related immunologically to AFP or CEA. It may be related to a 73,000 molecular weight protein (Ishii and Kanda, 1980) extracted from hepatoma tissues. This protein had a sedimentation coefficient of 6.3 and an isoelectric point of 9.3.

A Specific γ-Glutamyl Transpeptidase

A unique γ-glutamyl transpeptidase isoenzyme was demonstrated in hepatomas (Sawabu et al., 1983). This isoenzyme was present in 30% of cases where AFP levels were less than 400 ng/ml. Overall incidence was 55% of 200 hepatoma patients and only 7% of 279 patients with other hepatobiliary diseases. It was present in 52% of patients with Stage I disease. This isoenzyme is a useful marker for hepatomas. It is probably an oncofetal antigen. Although in many respects it was similar to the normal kidney enzyme, it differed in molecular weight, electrophoretic mobility, Con A affinity, sensitivity to neuraminidase, and isoelectric point (Toya et al., 1983).

A Retinoid-Binding Protein [CRBP(F)]

This isoenzyme is present in fish eye cytosol. By (^{3}H)-retinol binding assays it was demonstrated in 7 of 10 hepatomas (Muto and Omori, 1981). CRBP(F) is present also in human fetal liver and regenerating rat liver.

An Isoenzyme of Serum Ribonuclease With Acidic pI

This isoenzyme was detected in the serum of patients with hepatomas but not of those with diseases other than malignant neoplasms (Hishiki et al., 1984). It was detected also in the serum of patients with pancreatic carcinoma and in tissues of fetal liver and pancreas.

Tumor-Associated Markers

Thyroxine-binding globulin (TBG)

In patients with hepatomas as well as with metastatic carcinomas serum thyroxine-binding globulin (TBG) was elevated above normal levels in spite of there being no abnormalities of the thyroid gland (Terui, 1984). In conjunction with liver scintigrams, TBG was a good marker for evaluating liver with respect to the presence of tumors, especially metastases from other sites.

5'-Nucleotide phosphodiesterase isoenzyme (5'NPD-V)

This enzyme was found prominently present in six hepatomas examined histochemically (Tsou et al., 1982b). The tumor cells stained many times darker than the surrounding hepatocytes or the cells in cirrhotic areas. There was less evidence of AFP than CEA in the same tumor areas.

Serum ferritin

This tumor-associated marker cannot be used as an aid in differential diagnosis of hepatomas. It can be a useful marker in those cases where serum AFP levels are not elevated. Serum ferritin was found with a frequency of 97% in 35 hepatoma patients but also in 87% of 23 patients with cirrhosis (Melia et al., 1983).

Aldolase A

This isoenzyme which is present in small amounts in normal has been found to increase in the tumor cells of hepatomas. Serum adolase A was elevated in 94% of 34 patients with hepatomas and in all 29 with metastases, studied by Asaka et al. (1983). It was increased in more hepatoma patients than was serum AFP. In normal individuals serum adolase A was 171 $\pm$ 39 ng/ml (mean $\pm$ 2 SD).

Tumor-Specific Markers

Des-γ-carboxyl prothrombin is an abnormal prothrombin. It was found elevated (mean 900 ng/ml) in the serum of 91% (69 of 76) of patients with hepatomas (Liebman et al., 1984). This prothrommbin was not detected in normal individuals and was only slightly elevated (mean 10 ng/ml) in patients with chronic active hepatitis or metastatic carcinomas in the liver (mean 42 ng/ml). Thus, it may be useful marker for hepatomas.

As there is for breast and colon carcinomas, there is a tumor-specific β_2-microglobulin-associated antigen for hepatomas (Thomson et al., 1978). Evidence for tumor-specific hepatoma antigen has been reported also by use of leukocyte adherence inhibition assays (Morizane et al., 1980).

Further studies may confirm the preliminary suggestion that an alkaline-stable form of a cathepsin B-like compound occurs only in the sera of patients with hepatomas and not in the sera of those with acute hepatitis or cirrhosis (Dufek et al., 1984). This proteinase may be a marker for detection of early hepatoma developing in cirrhotic liver.

Viruses

In Korea hepatitis B virus (HBV) infection has been considered a major factor in the development of hepatomas. In all 112 hepatoma patients studied there was evidence of HBV infection, as well as in 97% of age- and sex-matched controls (Chung et al., 1983). It was determined that 87% of hepatoma patients were hepatitis B surface antigen (HBsAg)-positive, whereas only 14% of controls were positive for HBsAg. Hepatitis B antigen was not detected in 9 control individuals positive for HbsAg but was present in 38%

of hepatoma patients positive for HBsAg. While serum AFP was elevated in 83% of hepatoma patients, only 1 (1.5%) of 63 controls had elevated serum AFP.

Using assays to analyze immune complexes, Brown et al. (1984) observed that HBsAg can occur in an immune-complex form in the sera of patients classified as HBsAg-negative. Thus the incidence of HBV infection in association with hepatoma is greater than has so far established.

Since HBV infection is associated with the pathogenesis of hepatoma, a hypothesis was proposed to the effect that HBV infection early in life, transmitted by an HBV-carrier mother, leads to chronic active hepatitis, postnecrotic cirrhosis, and hepatoma (Hann et al., 1982). This hypothesis was supported by examining 664 first-degree relatives and 132 patients with chronic liver disease in Korea for the presence of HBsAg, antibodies to HBsAg, and antibodies to HBcAg. Mothers of the patients had a higher frequency of positive HBsAg than age-matched controls. Five fathers, 2 mothers and 5 brothers of patients had died of hepatoma.

There was a peculiar distribution of these markers as demonstrated histochemically in one 16-year-old hepatoma patient without evidence of acute or chronic liver disease (Gasser et al., 1983). The patient's serum contained HBsAg, HBeAg, antibody to hepatitis B core antigen, and 75 ng/ml AFP. Histochemically, the tumor cells contained mostly AFP and no HBsAg, and there was some CEA in tumor cells of lymph node metastases. HBsAg was present in nontumorous liver cells. A similar observation was made studying 150 autopsy cases (Kawano, 1983). The HBsAg-positive cells were the hepatocytes among the tumor cells. HBsAg-positive cells were not present in tumor thrombi in portal veins or pulmonary metastases.

DNA of HBV was integrated into the DNA of the hepatomas of 10 cases examined by Hino et al. (1984). There was no integration of HBV DNA in hepatomas of patients without HBV markers in the serum or tissues.

Fibrolamellar Carcinoma (FLC)

This tumor is a recently recognized variant of hepatoma. A highly characteristic marker for FLC is vitamin B_{12}-binding capacity (Paradinas et al., 1982). In 10 FLC cases there was no increase of serum AFP above normal levels. The tumor cells contained copper, copper-binding protein, and α_1 antitrypsin (Vecchio et al., 1984). In many respects FLC resembles focal nodular hyperplasia and appears to be a malignant counterpart of it.

Cholangiocarcinomas

There are fewer cholangiocarcinomas than hepatomas, and fewer tumor markers have been studied for this type of liver tumor. A tumor-associated antigen, CA19-9, was found increased above 37 U/ml in the serum of 73% of patients with cholangiocarcinoma (Jalanko et al., 1984).

KIDNEY TUMORS

Fetorenal Antigen

Fetorenal antigen was detected in epithelia of intra- and extrarenal excretory ducts and the urinary bladder (Kistler and Sonnabend, 1974). It cross-reacted immunologically with hepatitis B antigen. With immunofluorescence microscopy, antibodies to fetorenal antigen were found in all 15 cases of patients with renal carcinomas. These patients had no immunoelectrophorectically demonstrable hepatitis B antigen or antibodies to it.

Tumor-Associated Antigens

An antigen with a molecular weight of less than 70,000 was isolated from a renal cell carcinoma by Wright et al. (1977). Using the lymphocyte migration inhibition assay, they found that reactivity against this antigen was significantly greater with lymphocytes from renal cell carcinoma patients than with cells from patients with other conditions or from healthy subjects.

Three types of renal carcinoma cell surface antigens have been defined using autologous sera (Ueda, 1983): individually distinct antigens, shared tumor antigens, and normal cell surface antigens. Of 17 monoclonal antibodies to renal carcinoma cell lines none was tumor-specific.

Serum Haptoglobin (SH)

SH was found elevated in 58% of 116 patients with renal cell carcinoma (Babian and Swanson, 1982). The levels of SH correlated with the tumor burden and reflected the clinical course. They were elevated in about 13% of individuals without renal cell carcinoma. In spite of the low specificity as a tumor-associated marker, SH can be an indicator for the clinical surveillance of renal cell carcinoma.

Ferritin

High ferritin concentration in serum and in tissues has been noted in patients with renal cell carcinomas (Andersen, 1979). The renal cell carcinoma ferritin species was the most cathodic precipitate on rocket-immunoelectrophoresis. Basic isoferritin was present at high concentration in a case with renal cell carcinoma associated with hypercalcemia (Mufti et al., 1982). After removal of the tumor, calcium and ferritin levels returned to normal.

Tumor-Specific Markers

Markers for Renal Cell Carcinoma

There is a specific antigen in renal cell carcinoma, as shown by Teichman and Vogt (1974). It was demonstrated by a rabbit antiserum to pooled renal carcinoma tissues. After repeated absorption with normal tissues, the antiserum reacted specifically with renal cell carcinoma only. ^{131}I-labeled antiserum localized in the metastases, thus making it possible to detect these sites. A similar technique for localizing renal cell carcinoma was used with ^{131}I-labeled specific goat antibody to this tumor (Belitsky et al., 1978). Specific antigen was also demonstrated with a monoclonal (S25) antibody (Ueda et al., 1981).

Wilms Tumor Antigen

A specific antigen (W) has been demonstrated with an antiserum to Wilms tumor (Burtin and Gendron, 1973). This antigen is a glycoprotein. Although immunologically related, it was chemically different from bovine fetuin (Allerton et al., 1976). In another study (Waghe and Kumar, 1977) a monospecific antiserum to Wilms tumor failed to cross-react with fetuin.

Viruses

There were virus-like particles in three papillary carcinomas of renal pelvis studied by Elliott et al. (1973). Whereas particles resembling type A were detected in normal kidney tissues, type C was found only in tumors. Tumor cell cultures produced infective type C viruses. The patients' sera had neutralizing antibodies against viruses from two tumors. The nature of these particles is not known.

TUMORS OF THE URINARY BLADDER

Oncofetal Markers

The oncofetal markers CEA (Zimmerman and Wahren, 1976) and HCG (Cabnal et al., 1981) were found to occur at above normal levels in the sera of bladder cancer patients with a frequency of 60% and 22%, respectively. However, in another study of 26 patients with transitional cell carcinoma, there was elevated CEA concentration in urine but not in serum (Jakse et al., 1983). Histochemically, CEA was demonstrated in the tumor cells.

CEA

It was found that if the urinary CEA concentration initially was above 30 ng/ml, the patients had a poorer prognosis than those with pretreatment levels below 30 ng/ml (Wahren et al., 1982). Decreasing CEA levels after treatment also indicated a better prognosis than that for patients with increasing CEA concentrations in urine. A high CEA concentration may indicate more frequent monitoring and more intensive treatment. The highest degree of prognostic accuracy was achieved by combining four parameters in the evaluation: T class, grade, urinary CEA before treatment, and cytopathological examination 4 months after treatment (Nilsson et al., 1981). The prediction of a recurrence-free interval could be well established by combining urinary CEA and cytology studies. Grade alone was less correlated with the prognosis than were T class or urinary CEA.

TPA

Urinary TPA was elevated significantly in patients with bladder carcinomas studied by Kumar et al. (1981) but the sample had to be collected over a 24-hr interval. The concentration of TPA in 2-hr samples was variable and did not correlate with the condition of the patient. TPA was found to be more sensitive than CEA for bladder cancers (Oehr et al., 1981). For TPA at a specificity of 95%, the sensitivity was 93%.

Tumor-Associated Markers

Antigen Deletion

Deletion of ABH blood group antigens in bladder carcinomas is well known. The T antigen, a precursor of certain blood group antigens (Thomsen-Friedenreich antigen) appeared as a prognostic indicator in tumors with blood group ABH antigen deletion (Coone et al., 1982). Loss of T antigen was associated with 67% invasion, while only 17% of the tumors became invasive if cryptic T antigen was present, unmasked by treatment with neuraminidase.

There was good overall correlation between the deletion of ABH antigens and the behavior of bladder tumors in a study by Hofstadter and Jakse (1982). Among the patients with well-differentiated superficial tumors there were 8 deeply infiltrating recurrences in 12 cases with deleted ABH antigens, whereas no recurrent tumors were found in 18 patients with those antigens present. There was also a correlation with histologic grading. ABH antigens were present in 40% of grade 2, 8.5% of grade 3, and 0% of grade 4 carcinomas. Loss of the antigen occurred early in the development of the tumors. Expression of CEA by the tumor did not correlate with stage, grade, or clinical course as the pattern of the ABH antigens (Wiley et al., 1982).

This subject needs more investigation. In another study the absence of ABO (H) antigens did not correlate with histologic grading and could not predict poor prognosis (Nakatsu et al., 1984). On the other hand, CEA in the tumor tissues reflected the histologic grade and the survival rate.

Various Antigens and Glycosaminoglycans

Among four markers—chromosome mode, marker chromosomes, expression of the blood isoantigens, and Thomsen-Friedenreich antigen—the best indicator for Grade II carcinoma patients at risk for developing invasion was found to be the abnormal expression of Thomsen-Friedenreich antigen (Summers et al., 1983).

Several antibodies to urinary antigens of bladder cancer patients reacted with a frequency of 66% and with 25% in control individuals (DeFazio et al., 1982). Elevated excretion of urinary glycosaminoglycan has been noted in 53% of cancer patients (Hennessey et al., 1981). All 12 patients with metastases had elevated values.

Tumor-Specific Markers

Using lymphocytotoxicity microassays (Bubenik, 1975) or appropriately absorbed heterologous antisera to bladder carcinoma (Bloom, 1977), there was some evidence of an antigen specific for transitional cell carcinoma of the urinary bladder. Some such antigens may be represented by soluble membrane components (Hollinshead et al., 1979). There is also some evidence (O'Brien et al., 1980) that bladder tumor-specific antigens in urine are lower-molecular-weight components than antigens in urine from normal individuals or from patients with urinary tract infections.

A monoclonal antibody species to urinary β-glycoprotein was found to be selectively binding at the cell membranes of a transitional cell carcinoma (Hull et al., 1984). These antibodies did not bind to several normal cell types. If further studies of urine specimens reveal similar binding patterns, this antiserum may be a useful marker to identify malignant urothelial cells. Other monoclonal antibodies raised against human bladder transitional cell carcinoma were sufficiently specific to distinguish between normal transitional cells and transitional cell carcinomas (Messing et al., 1984).

Oncogenes

A cell line from human bladder carcinoma has been found to contain an oncogene c-H-*ras*-1 that differed from the normal cell oncogene by a point mutation and was a homologue of Harvey sarcoma virus *ras* gene (Parada et al., 1982). The product of this mutated gene was p21 altered at position 12 by substitution of glycine with valine, thus corresponding with DNA single-nucleotide change from G to T (Tabin et al., 1982). This alteration of p21 at position 12 has also been observed in products of c-K-*ras*-2 oncogenes in lung (Nakano et al., 1984) and colon carcinomas (Feinberg et al., 1983). The frequency of this specific tumor marker in bladder as in other carcinomas is not known. Altered p21 was not found in 29 patients with bladder, lung, or colon carcinomas (Feinberg et al., 1983).

Carcinoma of the Urachus

In 1 of 2 cases plasma CEA was elevated and it was useful in the follow-up during the clinical course (Saiki et al., 1982). The tumor was a mixed type mucinous adenocarcinoma and squamous cell carcinoma.

PROSTATIC CARCINOMAS

Serum CEA was found elevated in 40% of patients with prostatic carcinomas (Catalano and Menon, 1981). Tissue CEA was demonstrated in 50% of 10 grade I adenocarcinomas, 92% of 12 grade II carcinomas, 93% of 14 grade III carcinomas, and 93% of 15 tumors from patients with bone metastases (Ghazizadeh et al., 1984). Only 17% of 30 benign lesions had focal weak immunoperoxidase staining. Thus it appears that prostatic carcinomas produce CEA with great frequency, but the serum levels do not always reflect this production.

Tumor-Associated Markers

Prostatic Tissue-Specific Antigen

This tissue-specific antigen is a glycoprotein with a molecular weight of approximately 33,000 (Wang et al., 1977). With an enzyme immunoassay, it was found to be a useful marker for detecting prostatic carcinoma (Kuriyama et al., 1980). Its serum concentration correlated with the surgical stage of disease and the development of metastases (Pontes et al., 1982).

Acid Phosphatase Isoenzymes

Acid phosphatase has been used as a tumor marker of prostatic carcinoma. The prostatic isoenzyme is a glycoprotein with a molecular weight of about 100,000 (Chu et al., 1975) consisting of 7% carbohydrate and 93% protein.

This so-called prostatic acid phosphatase (PAP) is associated with prostatic carcinoma and appears in patients' serum at an increased concentration compared with normal individuals. The prostatic isoenzyme may not be elevated in sera of all patients with prostatic carcinoma (M.K. Gupta et al., 1981) and may be elevated in patients with nonprostatic cancer and benign prostatic hyperplasia.

At the earliest stages of prostatic adenocarcinoma the PAP was elevated only in 24% of patients (Griffiths, 1982). In stage C and stage D sera PAP was elevated in 75% and 100% of patients, respectively (Franchimont et al., 1983). However, PAP is an excellent marker for follow-up of patients during and after therapy, in spite of false-positive values in patients without carcinoma, e.g., with prostatitis (Van Cangh et al., 1982). PAP activity was also observed in neutrophils, and it can occur at an elevated level in the serum of patients with granulocytic leukemia (Yam et al., 1981). There are irregular fluctuations of serum enzyme levels (Brenckman et al., 1981). This should be taken into account during serial measurements to evaluate the effects of treatment or the course of the disease.

Parallel to PAP, there were found elevated serum levels of tissue polypeptide antigen in the sera of patients with prostatic carcinomas (Huber et al., 1983).

In those cases where PAP is not elevated, a useful adjunct marker for follow-up of patients was found to be creatine kinase isoenzyme CK-BB (Huber et al., 1982). As a marker by itself, this isoenzyme does not contribute anything else to the measurement of PAP. With a new immunoradiometric assay using a dual monoclonal antibody reaction system (Davies and Gochman, 1983), clinically undetected stage I disease was detected in 44% of 9 patients.

As in other malignant neoplasms, there was absence of blood group antigens in prostatic carcinoma cells, using the specific red blood cell adherence test (Walker et al., 1984). This test may be valuable in differential diagnosis of some atypical prostatic lesions with the exception of blood type O patients. In come of these patients the reaction was negative in normal and hyperplastic foci of the prostatic epithelium.

Prostaglandins

Prostaglandin 6-keto-$PGF_{1\alpha}$ was elevated in plasma of patients with prostatic cancer reported by Khan et al. (1982). This prostaglandin was more effective than prostatic acid phosphatase in detecting early stages of disease. It was useful also in the follow-up of patients during and after treatment.

Hydroxyproline

Urinary hydroxyproline excretion was found to be an important and sensitive marker for response to therapy when metastases involved bone (Hopkins et al., 1983).

Tumor-Specific Markers

Prostatic carcinoma-specific antigens have been demonstrated with immunofluorescence microscopy (Ablin et al., 1974), the leukocyte migration inhibition method (Wright et al., 1978), and use of monoclonal antibodies (Wright et al., 1981). One antigen in prostatic tissues with carcinoma specificity was demonstrated with an antiserum to carcinoma tissues using immunodiffusion techniques (Wang et al., 1977) or immunoperoxidase microscopy (Nadji et al., 1981b).

PCA-1 is an antigen with a molecular weight of approximately 40,000 that is highly specific for prostatic carcinomas (Edwards et al., 1982). Urine from prostatic carcinoma patients only contained this marker. A monoclonal antibody, 83.21, was also highly specific for prostatic carcinomas (Starling et al., 1982). It reacted with cytomegalovirus-transformed human embryonic lung cell line but not with normal embryonic cells.

Both these antigens can be potentially sensitive and specific markers for prostatic carcinomas.

Virus-like Components

C-type particles (Dmochowski and Ohtsuki, 1979), interspecies p30 (Kouttab et al., 1978), and reverse transcriptase (Arya et al., 1976) have been demonstrated in prostatic carcinomas. Herpesvirus type 2 antigens were demonstrated in prostatic tissues of 5% of 305 patients with benign prostatic hypertrophy and carcinoma (Baker et al., 1981). Significantly more patients with carcinoma had antibodies to herpesvirus type 2 than did patients with benign hypertrophy.

Adenoid Cystic Carcinoma of the Prostate

Adenoid cystic carcinoma, a rare tumor of the prostate, does not contain the two markers prostatic-specific acid phosphatase and prostatic-specific antigen (Kuhajda and Mann, 1984).

Immunoradiodiagnosis

^{131}I-labeled antibody against PAP has been used to localize metastatic tumor (Goldenberg et al., 1983b). Total-body photoscans with a γ-scintillation camera revealed primary and metastatic sites in two patients tested. This technique, using tumor markers, can be improved if the markers used are highly specific for a given neoplasm or universally for any malignant growth.

TUMORS OF THE FEMALE GENITAL TRACT

Tumor-associated trypsin inhibitor (TATI) is related to pancreatic secretory trypsin inhibitor and can be used to discriminate various gynecologic malignant neoplasms from nonmalignant gynecologic disease (Huhtala et al.,

1983). Elevated urinary TATI above an internal reference value of 7–50 μg/g creatinine was observed in 53% of 148 patients with gynecologic malignant neoplasms. In the reference population, which consisted of 98 patients with nonmalignant diseases and 40 with severe inflammatory or infectious diseases, the median urinary concentration of TATI was 22 μg/g creatinine. Cervical carcinoma patients had the highest urinary TATI levels.

α-L fucosidase activity was found to be increased in tumor tissues of endometrial, cervical, and ovarian carcinomas compared with corresponding normal tissues (Visce and Biondi, 1983). This enzyme inhibits macrophage migration and thus can contribute to uncontrolled growth of the neoplasms.

Vaginal Carcinoma

The etiology of verrucous carcinoma of the vagina may be associated with human papillomavirus (Okagaki et al., 1984). Type 6 HPV DNA was detected in two patients with this carcinoma. No structural protein was detected, but virus-like particles were observed by electron microscope in one case.

Carcinomas of the Vulva

Cysteinyl protease activity could be used as a marker for carcinomas of the vulva or vagina. However, it had a low sensitivity and specificity. The enzyme activity in urine was elevated in only 45% of patients with these carcinomas (Perras et al., 1983). About 40% of patients with nonmalignant diseases and pregnant women at term also had elevated urine enzyme levels.

Herpes Simplex Virus

Herpes simplex virus type 2 (HSV-2)-specific proteins were detected in the majority of squamous cell carcinomas *in situ* of the vulva according to Kaufman et al. (1981). Antibodies to HSV-2 were present in sera of 9 patients with this kind of tumor and in 2 healthy individuals. It appeared that infection with HSV-2 could be associated with the development of intraepithelial carcinoma. Although VP143, an early nonstructural polypeptide of HSV-2, and VP119, the major envelope glycoprotein, were demonstrated in some severe dysplasias, carcinomas *in situ*, and invasive squamous cell carcinomas (Cabral et al., 1982), there was no evidence of viral capsid proteins or virus particles. No infectious virus was isolated by cocultivation. It appeared that only a fragment of the viral genome was expressed.

Carcinoma of the Uterine Cervix

CEA

Serial CEA determinations have been found to reflect the course of the disease when it was in an early stage (Kjorstad and Orjasester, 1982). Patients with plasma levels higher than 5 ng/ml developed recurrent disease at a rate of 65% after initial therapy for stage IB squamous cell carcinoma. Furthermore, during the follow-up of many cases CEA levels increased before there was other clinical evidence of the recurrence of the carcinomas. In addition, immunohistochemically the pattern of the CEA in the lesions was different for invasive and noninvasive carcinomas (Bychkov et al., 1983). Invasive tumor contained CEA-positive cells at the stromal junction of the epithelial layer. This was not seen in noninvasive lesions.

cGMP-to-cAMP Ratio

With the routine screening of women with periodic cytological examination the incidence of invasive squamous cell carcinoma of the cervix has decreased considerably from the period of prescreening some 30 years ago. However, there are so-called premalignant lesions or cervical intraepithelial neoplasia (CIN), which is detected with considerable frequency. A biochemical marker for this CIN grade III is the ratio of urinary cyclic nucleotides—cyclic guanosine 3′:5′-monophosphate (cGMP) to cyclic adenosine 3′:5′-monophosphate (cAMP). In patients with severe dysplasia or carcinoma *in situ* (CIN III) the cGMP:cAMP ratio in urine was above 0.2 (Duttagupta et al., 1982). The ratio fell significantly after surgical treatment. This marker may prove valuable in the monitoring of patients, along with cytological studies.

Various Proteins

Plasma histaminase activity was found significantly higher in patients with squamous cell carcinoma than in controls (Birdi et al., 1984). the plasma enzyme level reflected th effects of radiotherapy.

Cysteinyl protease activity in urine was elevated in 78% of 32 patients with cervical carcinoma reported by Perras et al. (1983). It was elevated also in about 40% of patients with nonmalignant disease and pregnant women at term.

The urinary peptide 6K was found in 71% of 14 patients with cervical carcinoma (Stenman et al., 1982). This peptide is also elevated in other malignant neoplasms of the female genital tract and in amniotic fluid.

An Antigen in Squamous Cell Carcinoma of the Uterine Cervix (TA-4)

TA-4 is a glycoprotein with a molecular weight of approximately 48,000 (Kato et al., 1979). This marker is produced by squamous cell carcinoma of the cervix at a significantly higher rate than by normal stratified squamous epithelium of the cervix. The difference in TA-4 production is reflected in the serum. Thus, this antigen is a useful marker for evaluating the clinical course of the disease. Perhaps an antigen detected by heterologous cervical carcinoma antiserum (Haines et al., 1981) is related to this glycoprotein. The prognosis was found to be worse if the TA-4 was markedly elevated and the percentage of lymphocytes in the total leukocyte counts of the peripheral blood was less than 30.

Various Tumor-Associated Antigens

Heterologous serum raised to fractions of cervical carcinomas reacted with an antigen in the serum of 75% of 36 patients with cervical carcinoma, 6% of 8 with other gynecological diseases, and 1 of 72 pregnant women reported by Adelusi (1982). This antigen was not detected in 36 healthy controls by gel immunoprecipitation.

In addition, it was demonstrated by Bashford and Gough (1983) that the serum of patients with dysplasia contained a factor with a molecular weight of approximately 50,000 that significantly inhibited high-affinity rosette formation with normal lymphocytes. The patients with intraepithelial carcinoma contained two more such factors, with molecular weights of 73,000 and 88,000. No such factors were detected in stage I invasive squamous cell carcinomas.

As in many neoplasms, it was found that there was also a loss of blood group antigens in condyloma acuminata (Mambo, 1983). It occurred at a frequency of 80%. It is not known whether these lesions with the loss of blood isoantigen represent a group at risk of malignant transformation and those with isoantigens represent a group with regression of epithelial abnormalities.

A monoclonal antibody, OKT9, raised against an epitope of transferrin receptor was associated with the antigen in cervical dysplasias (J.M. Lloyd et al., 1984). Histochemically the binding of OKT9 to marked dysplasia was more pronounced and was not observed in slight dysplasias or normal epithelium. Basal layer cells of normal epithelium occasionally were associated with this antibody.

A specific antigen in cervical carcinoma has been demonstrated using rabbit antiserum to pooled carcinoma tissues (Teichmann and Vogt, 1974). After extensive absorption with various tissues, this antiserum reacted only with cervical carcinoma.

Viruses

Papillomavirus (PV) and Cervical Dysplasia

By immunoperoxidase microscopy, PV antigens were demonstrated in 48% of cervical dysplasias and 50% of vulvar condylomas. These viruses may be associated with the development of such lesions (Kurman et al., 1981). Since both PV antigens and DNA sequence in nuclei of atypical cells were demonstrated in 5 of 8 cases with mild dysplasia (Kurman et al., 1982), it was suggested that these lesions be segregated from unspecified dysplasias and designated as "papilloma-virus infection of the cervix". In 28 biopsy specimens with presence of immunohistochemically demonstrable PV internal capsid antigen, there were typical koilocytic cells and cytoplasmic maturation with atypical nuclei (Dyson et al., 1984). PV antigens were demonstrated in all papillomatous lesions and in none of the noncondylomatous dysplasias (Syrjanen et al., 1983a). However, using antiserum to genus-specific antigen, PV antigen was demonstrated in 43% of 152 cases with mild, 15% of 82 with moderate, and 17% of 47 with severe dysplasia, and in 10% of 41 with intraepithelial carcinomas. It was suggested that this decrease in the PV antigens in more advanced lesions was a result of eventual incorporation of the virus into the host DNA and nonexpression of the antigens (Syrjanen and Pyrhonen, 1982).

Herpes simplex virus type 2 (HSV-2)

It appears (Aurelian et al., 1981) that an antigen designated ICP 10/AG-4 may be a virus-encoded protein related to maintenance of a transformed phenotype. Antibodies (IgM) to this antigen were detected in increasing frequencies in the sera of patients with dysplasia, intraepithelial carcinomas and invasive carcinomas of the cervix. The antigen, or antibodies to it, can serve as markers for monitoring the effects of treatment. When cervical biopsy tissues were examined by *in situ* hybridization to DNA of herpes simplex virus (Eglin et al., 1981), HSV-specific RNA was detected in 72% of intraepithelial carcinomas, 60% of squamous cell carcinomas, 9% of adenocarcinomas of the cervix, and 2% of non-neoplastic tissues. This RNA was not associated with an overt HSV infection.

An early nonstructural polypeptide (VP143) of HSV-2 was present in 31% of marked cervical dysplasias, 29% of intraepithelial carcinomas, and 41% of invasive squamous cell carcinomas reported by Cabral et al. (1983). Evidently only a portion of the HSV-2 genome was expressing VP143 in the cells. There was no evidence of the major capsid protein or viral particles.

Adenocarcinoma of the Cervix

CEA was detected in 64% of 14 adenocarcinomas of the cervix studied by Speers et al. (1983). On the other hand 95% of 2 microglandular benign hyperplasias contained no immunohistochemically demonstrable CEA.

Endometrial Carcinomas

It has been found that in some uncertain cases it is possible to differentiate endometrial carcinoma from cervical adenocarcinoma by use of CEA. While CEA content estimated immunohistochemically was present in cervical adenomas, with the exception of squamous metaplasia, it was not present in endometrial carcinoma cells (Ueda et al., 1983).

Cysteinyl protease activity was elevated in the urine of 72% of 32 patients with endometrial carcinoma (Perras et al., 1983). The activity of this enzyme was also elevated in other patients with gynecological malignancies and in about 40% of patients with noncancerous disease as well as in pregnant women at term. A urinary peptide (OK) was present at an increased concentration in the serum of 64% of 14 patients with endometrial carcinomas reported by Stenman et al. (1982).

Ovarian Carcinomas

Oncofetal Markers

A unique antigen present in ovarian carcinomas has been found to cross-react with antigen in fetal and neonatal serum (Kalashnikov et al., 1976). This antigen was characterized by rabbit antisera to extracts of ovarian adenocarcinomas, using immunodiffusion and immunoelectrophoresis methods.

With rabbit antisera to ovarian cystadenocarcinomas, six antigens were identified (Imamura et al., 1978). One of them, OvC-6, was an individually specific antigen, which could be detected only in the tumor used for immunization. There are two types of ovarian cystadenocarcinomas: serous and mucinous. It may well be that these tumors differ antigenically. The other ovarian carcinomas—granulosa cell tumors—have antigens that can be distinguished from those of cystadenocarcinomas (Bhattacharya et al., 1979).

The antigen OCAA apparently is associated with ovarian carcinomas and is also present in the serum of pregnant women (Bhattacharya and Chatterjee, 1980). It is glycoprotein and can be readily detected by radioimmunoassay in the sera of patients with ovarian carcinomas. It is common to all cystadenocarcinomas of the ovary. A specific antigen for serous cystadenocarcinoma has also been demonstrated (Bhattacharya and Barlow, 1973). Its relationship to fetal tissues is not known.

In 15 mucinous cystadenocarcinomas the tumor markers pregnancy-specific β_1-glycoprotein (SP1) and placenta-specific tissue proteins (PP5, PP10, PP11, and PP12) were distributed as follows: PP5, 80%; PP11, 66.7%; SP1, 53.3%; PP12, 46.7%; and PP10, 20.0%. In 20 serous cystadenocarcinomas the distribution was PP5, 76.2%; PP11, 57.1%; SP1, 35%; PP12, 23.8%;

and PP10, 9.5% (Inaba et al., 1982). These markers can be applied to the monitoring of patients with ovarian carcinomas.

The most common universal oncofetal markers—CEA, AFP, and HCG—were found elevated in the serum of ovarian carcinoma patients at a rate of 57% (Khoo et al., 1982), 19% (Kizawa et al., 1983), and 40% (Vaitukaitis et al., 1976), respectively. Serum AFP was elevated in two patients with mixed mesodermal tumors (Blumkenfeld et al., 1984).

CEA

Serum CEA values have been found to correlate with those of ascitic fluid but not those of cyst fluid and tumor tissues. Serum CEA values were lower than CEA concentrations in the three other sites (Khoo et al., 1982). CEA in ascitic fluid was above 5 ng/ml in 43% of cases where serum CEA was below this level.

Liver metastases were predicted correctly in 86% of patients when serum CEA levels exceeded 10 ng/ml and this measurement was combined with liver scanning employing technetium colloid (Sonnendecker et al., 1984).

CA125

About 80% of patients with ovarian carcinomas have an antigen (CA125) in the tumor tissues that reacts with a murine monoclonal antibody, OC125, according to Kabawat et al. (1983). This antibody also reacted with amnion and derivatives of coelomic epithelium. In addition it reacted with mesotheliomas, adenocarcinomas of the endocervix, endometrium, and oviducts, and 7 of 64 nongynecological tumors examined. In nonmalignant adult tissues the epithelia of oviducts, endocervix, endometrium, and mesothelia reacted with OC125.

OC125 has been produced against a cell line from a serous papillary cystadenocarcinoma. Using immunofluorescence flow cytometry and microscopy 6 ovarian carcinoma cell lines were found to react with OC125. Among cell lines of different malignant neoplasms only one cell line of melanoma reacted with this antibody. In addition 5 of 9 cryopreserved ovarian carcinomas were positive for the antigen recognized by OC125. This antibody did not cross-react with any normal adult tissues including one fetal lung. Evidently the antigen recognized by OC125 is highly specific for ovarian carcinomas; however, 2% of 960 healthy individuals and 4.5% of 131 patients with nonmalignant diseases had elevated levels of the corresponding antigen CA125 (Bast et al., 1983). This antigen was associated with nonmucinous ovarian carcinomas and supplemented CEA as a marker in follow-up studies.

6K peptide

A 6,000-dalton peptide has been detected by an antiserum to a peptide fraction of urine from an ovarian cancer patient (Stenman et al., 1982). This 6K peptide is present at 5–20 ng/ml concentration in the serum of healthy individuals. It was elevated in 5 of 8 patients with ovarian cancer, in other gynecologic carcinomas, and in amniotic fluid of 14–16 weeks pregnancy.

Placental alkaline phosphatase

The median levels of this isoenzyme were found to be 50 times higher in cyst fluid of patients with various carcinomas than in fluids of benign cysts (Doellgast and Homesley, 1984). Serum enzyme levels did not correlate with tumor burden. In some patients with metastases serum enzyme concentration was not increased above normal values. The prognosis, however, was poorer for those patients who at the time of cancer diagnosis had elevated serum placental alkaline phosphatase than for patients with normal values.

Tumor-Associated Markers

Among tumor-associated markers the ones most frequently elevated in serum were β-2-microglobulin, lactic dehydrogenase, and hydroxybutyrate dehydrogenase, with an incidence of 57%, 53%, and 46%, respectively (Kikuchi et al., 1984). When all these markers were measured for each patient, the frequency with which at least one was elevated was 85%. In stage I cases the incidence of one elevated marker was 64%.

Cyclic GMP

Urinary cyclic guanosine 3′:5′ phosphate concentration was a sensitive marker for follow-up of patients with ovarian carcinoma (Turner et al., 1982). Increased concentration occurred as much as 10 months before there was any clinical sign of recurrence.

Galactosyltransferase

Serum glycoprotein galactosyltransferase activity reflected tumor burden and clinical course in 60 patients followed up with serial determinations by Gauduchon et al. (1983).

Cysteinyl protease

Cysteinyl protease activity was found elevated in the urine of 80% of 20 patients with ovarian carcinomas (Perras et al., 1983). It was also elevated in 44% of 66 pregnant women at term, and in 42% of patients with noncancerous diseases.

Amylase

Ovarian serous carcinoma produced amylase that was different from pancreatic and salivary gland amylases according to Van Kley et al. (1981). It was present in large amount in the cystic fluid of the carcinomas.

Tumor-Specific Markers

Unique antigens have been demonstrated with antisera to tumor tissues (Rozen, 1974) and with autoimmune antibodies from peritoneal effusions (Dorsett et al., 1975).

Heterologous antiserum to cyst fluid of a papillary mucinous cystadenocarcinoma, after appropriate absorption with normal tissues, reacted with mucinous cystadenocarcinoma, with borderline mucinous lesions, and with gastric and rectal carcinomas (Negishi et al., 1984), when tested with immunohistochemical microscopy. This antigen had a molecular weight of 450,000 and was not present in serous cystadenocarcinomas or mesonephroid tumors.

NB/70K

Glycoproteins isolated from ovarian carcinomas were found to be unique in these tumors. A glycoprotein has been purified and used with radioimmunoassay in clinical evaluation of cancer patients (Knauf and Urbach, 1981). This unique antigen was designated NB/70K; it appeared to be a far better marker for ovarian carcinoma than other markers for evaluating the course of the disease.

Ascites fluid from patients with malignant tumors has been examined immunohistochemically using an antiserum against the 70,000-dalton polypeptide component of NB/70K (Bizzari et al., 1983). This antigen was expressed by tumor cells of all ovarian carcinomas examined, including 14 serous, 5 endometrial, 2 undifferentiated, and 2 clear cell types. NB/70K was also present in cells from 2 endometrial and 2 unknown primary carcinomas examined as well as in 3 of 9 breast carcinomas. As determined by density gradient centrifugation, the NB/70K was expressed with greater frequency by nonproliferating, eventually more differentiated, cells.

An improved serum radioimmunoassay has been developed for measuring NB/70K levels in the sera of patients (Knauf et al., 1984). The measurements obtained by this method were accurate and reproducible.

Oncogenes

K-*ras* oncogene was activated in the tumor cells of ovarian cystadenocarcinomas (Feig et al., 1984). There was no activated K-*ras* oncogene in normal cells of tumor-bearing patients. Similarly K-*ras* oncogene was involved in a lung carcinoma patient (Santos et al., 1984).

The Monoclonal Antibody F36/22

The monoclonal antibody F36/22 possesses a high degree of specificity for the high-molecular-weight glycoproteins of ovarian carcinomas (Croghan et al., 1984). Adenocarcinomas, as well as exfoliated tumor cells, reacted with F36/22. The mesothelial cells and normal ovarian tissues with the exception of a few ductal elements did not react with this antibody. Thus, F36/22 can be a useful histochemical marker for ovarian adenocarcinomas.

Yolk Sac Tumors

In 6 patients with this tumor serum AFP ranged from 2,500 to 100,000 ng/ml (Malyama et al., 1984). The AFP concentration decreased during chemotherapy, but the patients with stage III disease died 4–9 months after surgery. One patient with stage Ia tumor was well, had normal AFP serum levels, and had no recurrence for 4 years after treatment. However, there may be instances where an AFP-positive tumor, as a result of selective outgrowth and cloning, changes its biological characteristics and becomes AFP-negative (Damjanov et al., 1984). Thus a recurrent tumor may be present without elevated serum AFP.

In one study the hyaline globules in yolk sac tumors of ovary and also testis contained AFP, but some did not (Nakanishi et al., 1982). The latter globules contained electron microscopically observable fine filamentous structures.

There is a special entity of yolk sac tumors with hepatoid differentiation (Prat et al., 1982). AFP and α-antitrypsin were identified in 4 and albumin in 2 of 7 such tumors.

Dysgerminoma

Serum LDH has been found elevated in patients with ovarian dysgerminoma (Awais, 1983). It decreased significantly after treatment. This is a marker for follow-up of patients with ovarian dysgerminoma.

Immunoradiodiagnosis and therapy

^{131}I-labeled antibodies to CEA were injected into 4 ovarian and 4 colorectal carcinoma patients with advanced metastatic diseases by Ford et al. (1983). After the localization of the conjugates in 5 patients, vindesine-labeled antibodies to CEA were injected with 1.2–42 ng antibody linked to 24–1,800 μg of vindesine. There were no undesirable reactions in these patients. It appears feasible to use CEA as a target for immunoradiodiagnosis and therapy.

3

Germ Cell Neoplasms

AFP and HCG are now widely used to follow up patients with germ cell neoplasms. While tumor markers lacking specificity and sensitivity cannot be used in screening for or diagnosis of malignant neoplasms, AFP and HCG are exceptions. Since AFP is produced by yolk sac tumors and HCG by choriocarcinomas, the presence of these markers in tissues or in the serum of patients with germ cell neoplasms indicates the presence of either yolk sac or syncytiotrophoblast elements.

It is well established that the markers in the serum are related to production by corresponding tumors. A close correlation between tissue AFP and HCG levels and the serum levels of these markers has been reported (Fowler et al., 1983).

Serum lactate dehydrogenase (S-LDH) also meets the criteria for an effective tumor marker for germ cell neoplasms (von Eyben, 1983). It was found elevated above normal levels of 8 μkat/liter in 50% of patients with testicular germ cell neoplasms. As the disease progressed or regressed, 88% of 52 patients had a concomitant increase or decrease of S-LDH. At the time of orchiectomy, the testicular vein on the side of the tumor contained a higher concentration of S-LDH than was found in the peripheral blood. Similar changes were noted in the serum lactate dehydrogenase isoenzyme (S-LDH-1) levels. S-LDH-1 concentration correlated with the tumor volume. None of 27 patients with early seminoma (75% of 36) had elevated serum LDH, whereas 82% of 11 with advanced disease had abnormally high values, according to Robertson and Read (1982). Serum LDH has also been found elevated in patients with ovarian dysgerminomas (Awais, 1983).

The effects of therapy can be estimated by the changes in serum marker levels, decrease of the marker concentration to a normal level indicating successful treatment. In the study of the effects of chemotherapy it was found that estimation of the marker's half-life indicated the effectiveness of therapy. If the decay rates of the markers are prolonged during the first month of chemotherapy, the chemotherapy is ineffective (Lange et al., 1982a). For example, both markers HCG and AFP contributed in the evaluation of patient status with intracranial germ cell tumors (Gjerris et al., 1982). Serum AFP was elevated in 5 of 8 patients preoperatively and in none postoperatively. The marker values eventually decreased postoperatively in all patients examined.

Alkaline phosphatase has been demonstrated histochemically in cell membranes of seminomas and embryonal carcinomas but not in choriocarcinomas or mature teratomas (Beckstead, 1983). This marker may supplement classification of germ cell tumors. Serum placental alkaline phosphatase was elevated in 40% of 30 patients with active seminomas (Javadpour, 1983). In addition, serum γ-glutamyl transpeptidase was elevated in 33% and HCG in 20% of 30 such patients. By combining all three markers for testing, at least one was elevated in 80% of 30 patients with active seminomas. When several species of alkaline phosphatase were discriminated with monoclonal antibodies (Paiva et al., 1983), it was found that 4 of 7 seminomas, 3 of 7 embryonal carcinomas, and 1 yolk sac tumor contained placental alkaline phosphatase. In addition, 2 other seminomas and 4 other embryonal carcinomas from the same series contained placenta-like alkaline phosphatase. The latter enzyme was so designated because it did not react with all 6 monoclonal antibodies raised against the human placental alkaline phosphatase.

SEMINOMAS AND DYSGERMINOMAS

It has been generally considered that seminomas in male and dysgerminomas in female patients do not produce the common germ cell tumor markers AFP and HCG. However, there have been several cases where elevated serum AFP was associated with tumors diagnosed as pure seminomas (Raghavan et al., 1982). This indicates a differentiation from yolk sac carcinoma, which has been observed in xenografts of human germ cell tumors. Those cases of seminoma where metastases consisted of yolk sac tumor and resisted radiation therapy can be explained on the basis of differentiation from another type. On the other hand it is possible that radiation therapy induces a change in the tumor towards differentiation. A tumor in the pineal region has been suspected of being a germ cell neoplasm. Serum HCG and AFP levels were not elevated above normal values (Hokin et al., 1983). The tumor regressed with radiation therapy. Three months after therapy the tumor recurred and the serum AFP was markedly elevated. The tumor was then removed and appeared to be a typical yolk sac tumor.

Placental alkaline phosphatase is a suitable marker for seminomas (Lange et al., 1982b). Serum enzyme was elevated above the normal upper level of 1.85 ng/ml in 57% of 28 patients with active seminomas. When parallel serum HCG determinations were done, the frequency of elevated value of one or the other marker was 71%. The serum placental alkaline phosphatase was not elevated in 36 controls including 30 with inactive testicular tumors. Although HCG does not occur in seminomas and dysgerminomas without the presence of cells resembling syncytiotrophoblasts, there may be exceptions. In a case of an ovarian tumor histologically as pure dysgerminoma, HCG was elevated (Zarabi and Rupani, 1984). The HCG-producing cells were identified immunohistochemically as small stromal cells. Such stromal cell production of HCG may occur in other pure tumors of this kind.

EMBRYONAL CARCINOMAS

Elevated serum AFP could be present in 73% of patients with embryonal carcinomas (Kurman et al., 1977). Since AFP is produced by the cells of yolk sac tumors, embryonal carcinomas may contain such cell types. However, one should not assume that elevated serum AFP is present exclusively in these tumors. There is a case report (Pritchett and Skinner, 1984) that an unexplained increase of serum AFP levels persisted in a patient for 2 years without evidence of recurrence of a tumor after therapy. AFP can be produced by other than tumor cells, especially as a result of chemotherapy (Coppack et al., 1983).

HCG, the other common oncofetal tumor marker, can be used to monitor patients with embryonal carcinomas. It was present in above-normal levels in the sera of 50% of the patients with this tumor (Braunstein et al., 1973). In these tumors probably there were trophoblastic cells producing HCG.

F9 Antigens as Oncofetal Markers

F9 antigens have been expressed by a mouse teratocarcinoma cell line. They are present in sperm of mammals, including man (Jacob, 1977) but not in other adult cells. However, these antigens are expressed by human embryonal carcinoma cells (Holden et al., 1977), osteosarcoma cells, choriocarcinoma, and hydatidiform mole (Singh et al., 1982). A patient with choriocarcinoma had antibodies against BALB/c mouse testicular antigens of this type. A monoclonal antibody raised to 4- to 8-cell-stage zona-pellucida-free mice embryos reacted with human embryonal carcinoma cells as demonstrated immunohistochemically (Damjanov et al., 1982). However, monoclonal antibody to mouse embryonal carcinoma cell line F9 did not react with human embryonal carcinoma cells. It reacted with cells of human yolk sac tumor components in a human teratoma and two embryonal carcinomas.

Antibodies were present in the serum of patients with ovarian germ cell neoplasms, which reacted with the murine cells of the line F9 (Kawata et al.,

1983). These human antibodies reacted with the same glycopeptide antigen as the murine antibodies to F9. When the F9 cells were exposed to retinoic acid-induced differentiation, the antigen was reduced, indicating that it is a differentiation antigen.

TROPHOBLASTIC TUMORS

Oncofetal Marker—Human Chorionic Gonadotropin

The β subunit of human chorionic gonadotropin (β-HCG), a normal placental hormone, is an indicator of the presence of choriocarcinoma or tumor cells resembling trophoblasts. A serum level of β-HCG higher than 1 ng/ml in adult males is considered elevated (Moore et al., 1978). The increased levels of β-HCG are produced by syncytiotrophoblasts (Javadpour and Bergman, 1978). The frequency of the elevated serum β-HCG correlates with the presence of syncytiotrophoblastic elements in tumors, germ cell neoplasms of females and males. This marker is most useful in evaluating trophoblastic malignancies (Skinner and Seckinger, 1979). Another oncofetal marker, placenta-specific tissue protein (PP′2) was less suitable for the follow-up of the patients with trophoblastic disease (Than et al., 1983). Nevertheless, the serum concentration of PP′2 reflected closely the clinical course of the disease.

Prolactin

Using immunoperoxidase microscopy, prolactin was demonstrated in all cases of 15 hydatidiform moles, 6 invasive moles, and 7 choriocarcinomas (Lee et al., 1981). Thus, both chorionic gonadotropin and prolactin can be used as markers for trophoblastic tumors.

Pregnancy-Specific β_1-Glycoprotein (SPI)

When serum samples were eluted on columns of concanavalin A (Con A) Sepharose, some of the SPI was bound and some unbound to Con A (Koistinen et al., 1981). The unbound fraction of SPI was greater in the sera of patients with choriocarcinoma than in any normal-pregnancy patient. This difference in binding properties of SPI was suggested to be due to altered glycosylation in choriocarcinoma cases.

TERATOMAS

In 24 children with mature teratomas, serum AFP was within normal limits (Tsuchida and Hasegawa, 1983). It was elevated in 31 of 32 with malignant teratomas. Thus AFP can contribute to the differential diagnosis. HCG in addition to AFP was a suitable marker for the evaluation of 69 men with metastatic malignant teratomas (Newlands et al., 1938). If the initial HCG levels in serum were below 50,000 U/liter and AFP below 500 kU/liter 96% of 47 patients survived. With higher concentrations of these markers only 56% of 22 survived.

CEA and AFP were present in the tumor tissues of sacrococcygeal teratomas at a rate of 82% and 53%, respectively (Kuhajda and Taxy, 1983). This is a rare tumor occurring in female infants.

Virus-like Particles in Teratocarcinomas

Five teratocarcinoma cell lines produced particles resembling C-type retroviruses (Kurth et al., 1981). The origin of these particles and their role in tumor development are not known.

Immunoradiodiagnosis was attempted using ^{131}I-labeled antibodies to AFP. Tumors were localized by scanning in all patients with elevated serum AFP and in two others without elevated serum AFP (Bradwell et al., 1983).

4

Skin Tumors

Histochemical studies have revealed that CEA is produced by tumors of ectodermal tissues (Scurry and de Boer, 1983). It was detected in all squamous cell carcinomas, keratoacanthomas, and pure basal cell carcinomas studied but not in normal adult skin. The skin of 12- to 18-week-old fetuses contained CEA.

MELANOMAS

Oncofetal Markers

Only a small percentage of the sera of patients with melanomas contain elevated levels of the well-known universal markers. AFP was present at a frequency of 20% (Mihalev et al., 1976), and HCG at 10% (Braunstein et al., 1973). There are two antigens on the cell membranes of the melanoma cells, one shared by melanoma cells and the other by fetal fibroblasts (Stuhlmiller and Seigler, 1975). Antigens of the cell surface of cultured melanoma cells cross-reacted also with those of fetal skin in complement-dependent cytotoxic antibody studies (Fritze et al., 1976). In the group of membrane antigens of melanoma cells, there is evidence that some are shared by fetal melanocytes (Galloway et al., 1981), benign melanocytic disorders (Fox et al., 1981), and fetal brain (Jones et al., 1981). IgM antibody titers to this antigen correlated with the patients' prognosis; higher levels of IgM antibody were associated with longer disease-free intervals and survivals.

An oncofetal antigen was present in melanoma tissue extracts as indicated by leukocyte migration inhibition assays (Cochran et al., 1982). Only melanoma patients' leukocytes were inhibited by melanoma and first-trimester fetal extracts.

Among the human melanoma markers, there is one glycoprotein with a molecular weight of 94,000 (Morgan et al., 1981), also found in a cell strain of fetal melanocytes. In the fetal melanocytes, although immunologically identical, this glycoprotein had a molecular weight of 90,000. After the transformation of these melanocytes with SV40, they synthesized the glycoprotein with a molecular weight of 94,000. It is not known whether other than virus-induced transformation would be associated with such a change in this oncofetal glycoprotein. A monoclonal antibody against this antigen reacted also with normal human sera (Morgan and Reisfeld, 1982).

A melanoma-associated antigen p97 (Brown et al., 1981b) may be similar or related to the oncofetal glycoproteins. Using monoclonal antibodies to p97, five epitopes were defined (Brown et al., 1981a). This antigen is a monomeric sialoglycoprotein. Using immunohistochemistry, the p97 was localized in melanoma cells only, not in other types of adjacent cells (Tilgen et al., 1983). By electron microscope this antigen was seen at the cell membranes. It is structurally and functionally related to transferrin and its gene is located on chromosome 3 (Plowman et al., 1983). After prolonged exposure to monoclonal antibodies against p97 (Hellström et al., 1983) melanoma cells in the tissue culture continued to express p97.

A melanoma-associated antigen (MAA) was present also in cultured fetal cells. It is a glycoprotein with a molecular weight of approximately 120,000 (Smalley and Bystryn, 1978). This antigen and others were shed from the cell membranes, in association with membrane fragments, by an energy-independent process (Bystryn and Tedholm, 1981). From another study (Ishii et al., 1980), it appeared that the oncofetal antigen had a molecular weight of 90,000 and that another antigen with a molecular weight of 120,000 was group-specific in different melanoma cell lines.

There are also common neuroectodermal oncofetal antigens shared by melanoma, neuroblastoma, retinoblastoma, glioblastoma, and fetal brain that cross-react with hybridoma antibodies raised against melanoma cells (Liao et al., 1981). Another monoclonal antibody raised to a human melanoma cell line was more specific for melanomas (Liao et al., 1982). While reacting with fetal tissue homogenates, it did not cross-react with other tumors that were also of neuroectodermal origin. The antigen has a molecular weight of approximately 87,000. It is a glycoprotein lacking internal disulfide linkages (Khosravi et al., 1983). A monoclonal antibody 140.240 reacted with the epitope and the peptide portion of this glycoprotein (gp87). Another monoclonal antibody to melanoma cells (140.72) reacted with 19 of 22 melanomas, 6 of 15 carcinomas, and 10 of 11 tissue homogenates from different fetuses (Liao et al., 1983). The corresponding antigen in reactive melanoma cells was a substance with a molecular weight of 95,000–150,000 and in carcinoma cells in addition another entity, consistent with CEA.

A lower-molecular-weight glycoprotein (15,000 daltons) was isolated from fetal liver (Salinas et al., 1982). This glycoprotein contained 3% carbohydrate and was designated HOFA (human oncofetal antigen). Immune complexes found with this antigen in melanoma patients' sera correlated in size with the tumor burden.

A monoclonal antibody raised against a melanoma cell line reacted with 94% of 17 melanoma specimens from 13 patients (Khan et al., 1983). This antibody reacted also with a squamous cell carcinoma cell line and amnion cells. Thus it can be classified as an oncofetal marker. It did not react with other different normal or abnormal tissues.

Tumor-Associated Markers

A marker with a molecular weight between 40,000 and 60,000 occurred in the sera of patients with melanoma and was produced by melanoma cells (Copeman and Cooke, 1979). It was not a specific marker, since the protein was produced also by cells of benign dermatoses: halo nevus, vitiligo, and lichen planus. Apparently, these cells are altered melanocytes and it is possible that a genetic change is present in both melanoma cells and in melanocytes of benign dermatoses. A monoclonal and a polyclonal antibody to a melanoma-associated antigen (MAA) of 100,000 molecular weight were used to estimate serum MAA of melanoma patients (Morgan et al., 1984). The concentration of serum MAA reflected the tumor burden. There is also evidence (Hook et al., 1983) that human and swine melanoma cells have a common tumor-associated antigen, which was not expressed by mouse B16 melanoma cells. The nature of this antigen has not been determined.

S-100 Protein

This protein was a useful marker in identifying histochemically amelanotic melanomas (Nakajima et al., 1981). It was present in nevi also and was more evident in lesions with lesser pigment production. S-100 protein is produced by Schwann cells and is found in tumors derived from these cells and melanocytes (Stefansson et al., 1982). It is also present in neurofibromas, neurilemomas, granular cell myoblastomas, but not in malignant Schwannomas, neuroblastomas, or other carcinomas. It is not an exclusive marker for neuroectodermal tumors. S-100 was demonstrated immunohistochemically in chondro-and liposarcomas as well as in chondrocytes and adipocytes (Cocchia et al., 1983). In addition, S-100 was present also in plasmorphic adenomas of salivary glands, in chordomas, and in breast or other tumors corresponding to myoepithelial cells (Nakajima et al., 1982).

A marker that is reactive with a monoclonal antibody NK1C3 was present in all melanomas examined immunohistochemically (Mackie et al., 1984). It was present also in benign melanocytic lesions; therefore, it could not be useful in the differential diagnosis of these entities. NK1C3 was useful in identifying melanoma in metastatic tumors in skin, such as lymphomas and breast, gastrointestinal tract, and other undifferentiated carcinomas. In comparison with S-100 antibodies, NK1C3 was located on more cells.

Ferritin

Ferritin was insignificantly elevated in the serum only of patients with stage III disease (Luger et al., 1983). It increased as the disease progressed with metastases. In stages I and II the serum ferritin levels were within the normal range.

Sialic Acid

Sialic acid levels in serum and the size of the tumor as a common factor were consistent an indicator of the disease progress in certain stages of malignant melanomas (Silver et al., 1983). The risk of recurrence by 2 years was 12 times greater for patients with lesions greater than 1.75 mm and sialic acid concentration less than 2 μmol/ml than for those with tumors less than or equal to 1.75 mm and sialic acid levels less than or equal to 2 μmol/ml.

Tumor-Specific Markers

Many studies using immunofluorescence microscopy with auto antibodies or heterologous antisera (Morton et al., 1968; Lewis et al., 1973; A.Y. Elliott et al., 1973) pointed to the existence of specific antigens in melanomas. With this technique, it was shown that melanoma-specific antigens did not cross-react with normal choroidal melanocytes (Federman et al., 1974). Melanoma-specific antigenic activity was also demonstrated by fluorescence microscopy and hemagglutination methods (Van Alstyne, 1977).

Other approaches to study of melanoma-specific antigens have been immunodiffusion (Viza and Phillips, 1975), antibody-dependent cell-mediated cytotoxicity assays (Hersey et al., 1976), leukocyte migration inhibition assays (McCoy et al., 1975; Kerney et al., 1977), immune adherence assays (Shiku et al., 1976), and use of antisera (Suter et al., 1975; Dent et al., 1976; Vennegoor et al., 1977) or autoimmune sera (Embleton and Price, 1978) to cultured melanoma cells, of cutaneous delayed hypersensitivity reactions (Hollinshead, 1975), and of hybridoma-produced antibodies (Woodbury et al., 1980; Hellström, et al., 1981; Imal et al., 1981; Natali et al., 1981). A double-determinant immunoassay was developed to measure a human high-molecular-weight melanoma-associated antigen (Giacomini et al., 1983). Using monoclonal antibodies to the determinants of this antigen, it was found that 4 of 8 melanoma tissues contained the antigen by binding a monoclonal antibody. Such binding was not observed to normal tissues including skin, congenital, or blue nevi. With immunofluorescence microscopy this antigen was demonstrated in melanomas and not in normal tissues.

Melanoma-Specific Protein

This protein consists of polypeptide chains with molecular weights of 116,000, 26,000, 29,000, and 95,000 (Mitchell et al., 1981). The latter chain is attached by noncovalent interactions, while the two smallest chains are linked by disulfide bonds to the largest chain.

β_2-Microglobulin-Associated Protein

This unique gene product isolated from melanomas occurs only in these tumors (Thomson et al., 1978). Some of its physical characteristics are similar to those of specific antigens of breast and colon carcinomas and of hepatomas. This protein has a molecular weight of about 70,000 and consists of three subunits. It is associated with β_2-microglobulin and cross-reacts immunologically with HLA antigens. It is possible that this antigen along with β_2-microglobulin was one of the components in an enhanced antigen expression by interferon (Liao et al., 1980).

Glycoproteins

Melanoma-associated antigens were examined in tissue culture using monoclonal and polyclonal antibodies (Galloway et al., 1981). A glycoprotein with a molecular weight of 240,000 was specific for melanomas. Another glycoprotein with a molecular weight of 94,000 was present on fetal melanocytes.

A monoclonal antibody to a plasma membrane-enriched fraction from melanoma cells reacted with a glycoprotein of 250,000 molecular weight and a sulfated molecule greater than 400,000. The antigen was identified as a chondroitin sulfate type A/C proteoglycan. These specific proteoglycans were located on the surface of the melanoma cells (Harper et al., 1984).

It is not known whether an apparently specific antigen with a molecular weight of 80,000–150,000 isolated from melanoma cell membrane (Leong et al., 1978) has common components with fetal cells. Among melanoma-specific antigens there was a component with a molecular weight of 90,000 that was an oncofetal antigen (Ishii et al., 1980). A membrane antigen of melanoma free of antigenic cross-reactivity with fetal cells had a molecular weight of 13,000 (Stuhmiller et al., 1978), while those with 17,000, 25,000, and 48,000 molecular weights had oncofetal antigen properties. A detailed analysis of these glycoproteins is not yet available. Perhaps some of them are very similar. One such 65,000-dalton glycoprotein specific for human melanomas and murine B16 melanoma cells appeared similar but not identical to serum albumin with respect to amino acid composition and some of their sequences (Marchalonis et al., 1984).

Specific Lipoproteins

While most of the tumor markers are glycoproteins, there are some exceptions. An antigenic system (R24) defined by monoclonal antibodies to cell surface membrane antigens consisted of heat-stable glycolypids (Dippold et al., 1980). A tumor-associated antigen (TAA) (R.K. Gupta et al., 1981), a specific marker with a molecular weight of 180,000, might be lipoprotein.

A Ganglioside

A monoclonal antibody was directed to surface antigen of human melanoma cells (Nudelman et al., 1982). It was a ganglioside, identical to brain ganglioside GD3, but with longer-chain fatty acids. This antibody did not react with other gangliosides.

By adding a single O-acetyl group to a cell surface disialoganglioside GD_3, a specific marker was created, which was similar to one occurring on human melanoma cells (Cheresh et al., 1984). This marker was recognized on the melanoma cells by a monoclonal antibody.

Virus-like Components

Human melanomas contained particles resembling C-type viruses (Birkmayer et al., 1974b). In addition, the cells contained an RNA-instructed DNA polymerase resembling characteristics of that in RNA viruses. There was also a 70S RNA species.

Immunoradiodiagnosis

^{131}I-labeled mouse monoclonal antibodies and Fab fragments specific for p97 antigen were used to detect melanomas (Larson et al., 1983). In six patients examined 88% of 25 lesions larger than 1.5 cm were detected after injection of antibodies and scanning. There were no toxic risk effects,

WARTS

Human papilloma virus type 1 (HPV-1) type-specific antiserum reacted with 50% of 24 plantar warts and 11% of 35 common warts (Jenson et al., 1982b). The warts associated with HPV-1 contained more viral particles and were more aggressive than the warts with other HPV species. In another study (Laurent et al., 1982) HPV-1 was associated with 74% of 50 plantar warts, and 18% of 50 were associated with HPV-2.

SWEAT GLAND CARCINOMAS

CEA was demonstrated immunohistochemically in all four sweat gland carcinomas examined (Penneys et al., 1982). It was present in the cytoplasm of the tumor cells and in the lumina of the tumor acini.

TRABECULAR CARCINOMAS

Neuron-specific enolase, a tumor-associated marker for neuroendocrine neoplasms, was demonstrated immunohistochemically in 70% of 10 trabecular carcinomas with cutaneous metastases (Wick et al., 1983).

5

Sarcomas

Oncofetal gene products are expressed by sarcomas. A monoclonal antibody raised to a glycoprotein of human peripheral blood monocytes reacted with six sarcoma cell lines tested immunohistochemically (Azzarone et al., 1984). It reacted with human embryonic fibroblasts also, but not with those of adult origin.

ONCOFETAL MARKERS

Various sarcomas, with the exception of rhabdomyosarcomas, reacted with monoclonal antibodies raised to a glycoprotein of approximately 55,000 molecular weight (Pagè et al., 1984). Using immunohistochemical methods 85% of sarcoma tissues as well as human fetal tissues reacted with this antiserum. It may be a potential marker for the sarcomas.

In some instances a specific marker can be located in other tumor cells than those producing the marker. Myoglobin was detected histochemically in breast carcinoma, melanoma, and lymphoma cells (Eusebi et al., 1984). This occurred in tumor cells infiltrating skeletal muscle. Some of the myoglobin was phagocytized in macrophages, some by tumor cells. Such phagocytic appearance should be considered in interpreting the nature of a tumor.

A small percentage (24%) of patients with embryonal rhabdomyosarcoma had elevated serum levels of CEA (Helson et al., 1976). Serum CEA was elevated (10.2 and 17.8 ng/ml) in a patient with pseudomyxoma peritonei (Salki et al., 1982). In this case there were no abdominal symptoms, but dyspnea due to bilateral pleural metastases.

TUMOR-ASSOCIATED MARKERS

There is an antigen shared by different sarcomas (Drewinko et al., 1973) and a neurogenic sarcoma cell line. This antigen in the neurogenic sarcoma cell line reacted with antibodies in the sera of patients with different sarcomas as demonstrated with immunofluorescence microscopy. Since one serum of

18 normal individuals reacted with this antigen also, it is not a tumor-specific but a tumor-associated marker, appearing more frequently in sarcomas than in normal tissues.

A tumor-associated antigen was demonstrated in the urine of sarcoma patients by the use of complement fixation assays (Huth et al., 1984). Of 25 patients with recurrent tumors, 96% had reappearance of TAA in urine. There was no TAA in 92% of 25 patients who remained disease-free.

SARCOMA-SPECIFIC MARKERS

Apparently there are antigens that are cross-reacting only among different sarcomas, others that are limited to one kind of sarcoma, and still others that are unique for a patient with a sarcoma.

Sarcoma Cross-Reacting Antigens

Sera from patients with sarcomas cross-reacted with different sarcomatous tumor tissues (Priori et al., 1971; Moore et al., 1973) or with urine concentrates of sarcoma patients (Huth et al., 1981). Patients with different sarcomas had developed a cellular immunity to osteosarcoma cells (Cohen et al., 1973).

Specific Antigen in Neurogenic Sarcomas

Sarcoma-specific antigen in a human neurogenic sarcoma line (T_2 cells) was localized with immunoperoxidase electron microscopy (Lichtiger et al., 1976). The antigen was present on the cell membrane. The reacting antibodies were from the sera of patients with sarcomas.

Tumor Markers in Sarcomas of Fibroblastic-Histiocytic Origin

Most of the malignant fibrous histiocytomas (82%) contain α_1-antitrypsin and ferritin (54%) as observed with immunoperoxidase microscopy (Kindblom et al., 1982). None of the spindle cell type or myxoid variant contained α_1-antitrypsin. From these studies it appeared that α_1-antitrypsin is a good marker for histiocytic differentiation. Monoclonal antibodies have been produced that react with a high degree of specificity with sarcomas and fibroblast cell lines only (Feit et al., 1982). They did not react with all carcinoma cell lines tested.

A Fetal Fibrosarcoma Antigen (ANS-3)

Using an indirect immunofluorescence method it was observed that antiserum to a human cerebral glycoprotein (ANS-3) cross-reacted with fibrosarcoma cells and connective tissues of other neoplasms. It also cross-reacted with connective tissues of fetal skin and intestine (Delpech et al., 1978).

MARKERS FOR MYOGENIC TUMORS

Z-protein is a component specific in muscle cells. It is a protein with a molecular weight of 55,000. Using immunoperoxidase histology, it was demonstrated in different myogenic neoplasms with the following frequencies: in 2 of 2 cardiac rhabdomyomas, 5 of 5 leiomyomas, 9 of 10 leiomyosarcomas, and 15 of 18 rhabdomyosarcomas (Mukai et al., 1984). Among the latter group Z-protein was present in 5 of 5 pleomorphic, 7 of 9 embryonal, and 3 of 4 alveolar types. This marker was not present in 77 other kinds of neoplasms examined. Thus Z-protein can serve as a distinct marker for the differentiation of myogenic tumors from other neoplasms with similar morphological appearance.

OSTEOGENIC SARCOMAS

Osteogenic Sarcoma Antigens

Elevated CEA levels were present in the sera of 81% of the patients with this type of sarcoma (Cortes et al., 1977).

Using microcytotoxicity assays it was found that lymphocytes from osteosarcoma and other sarcoma patients, as well as some carcinoma patients, reacted with fetal periosteal fibroblasts in tissue cultures (Gangal et al., 1975). Serum from an osteosarcoma patient blocked the reactivity of lymphocytes from 5 of 6 sarcoma patients, but did not block the reactivity of normal individuals or patients with carcinoma. This indicates specific antigenicity common to fetal periosteal fibroblasts and sarcomas. In addition, tumor cell membrane antigens blocked sarcoma activities specifically (Agashe et al., 1977), indicating that there might be a cell type-specific embryonic antigen in addition to a common one. Antibodies to these fetal antigens have also been demonstrated in the sera of normal individuals (Thorpe and Rosenberg, 1977).

Specific Antigens in Osteogenic Sarcomas

Although osteogenic sarcomas cross-react with antibodies from patients with various other kinds of sarcomas, there are limited antigens also. After extensive absorption of antifetal antibodies, autoimmune sera of patients reacted only with osteogenic sarcoma cells. This reactivity was specific for autologous tumors, not cross-reacting with similar tumors from other patients (Thorpe and Rosenberg, 1978).

Using affinity column chromatography, a specific antibody was isolated from human osteogenic sarcoma (Tsang et al., 1980). Some specific antigens may be detected by the use of monoclonal antibodies (Toyama, 1983). Some of the antibodies produced against fresh osteosarcoma cells were highly specific for osteogenic sarcomas. Subsequently, several human lymphoblastoid cell lines were established from B lymphocytes from a patient with osteogenic sarcomas (Tsang et al., 1984). These cells produced antibodies specific to osteogenic sarcoma cell lines. They did not react with other cells.

Oncogene-Related Products

As in several malignant neoplasms, osteogenic sarcomas too may express oncogene products. This was observed in an osteogenic sarcoma-derived cell line, U-2 OS (Graves et al., 1984). Antiserum to platelet-derived growth factor (PDGF) precipitated several polypeptides from the sarcoma cells. In addition, the sarcoma cells secreted a 29,000-dalton protein that was similar to PDGF. It had been shown earlier that a compound identical to PDGF is expressed by the v-*sis*, the transforming gene of the simian sarcoma virus. It is possible that these transcripts of the human cellular homologue (c-*sis*) maintain the transformed state.

MARKERS FOR TUMORS OF ENDOTHELIAL CELL ORIGIN

Factor VIII-Related Antigen (VIII R-Ag)

This antigen is a marker for endothelial cells and occurs in various neoplasms of endothelial cell origin (Sehested and Hou-Jensen, 1981). Thus, such tumors as Kaposi's sarcoma can be readily identified (Guarda et al., 1982; Nadji et al., 1981a).

Ulex europaeus I Agglutinin

Lectin-Ulex europaeus I agglutinin is even a better marker for endothelial cell derivatives than VIII R-Ag (Miettinen et al., 1983). This lectin binds specifically to the endothelial cells. It is associated also with those endothelial cell sarcomas that were negative for VIII R-Ag.

VIRUS-LIKE COMPONENTS

Distribution of antibodies to human osteogenic sarcomas in patients and members of their families suggested that an infectious agent was associated with this tumor (Morton and Malmgren, 1968). Subsequently, this suggestion was strengthened by the observation that cell-free extracts of human osteogenic sarcomas induced sarcomas in hamsters and these hamster tumors reacted with human sarcoma-specific antisera (Reilly et al., 1972). Sarcomas, including osteosarcomas, contained in their polysome fraction an RNA that was homologous to RNA of the Rauscher leukemia virus (Kufe et al., 1972).

A human fibrosarcoma cell line, HT1080, expressed an antigen related to p30, a protein of RD114 baboon endogenous virus (Smith et al., 1977).

Rous sarcoma virus-related human cell endogenous protein pp 60c-*src* kinase activity was increased fourfold to 20-fold in 3 of 9 sarcomas compared with normal tissues (Jacobs and Rubsamen, 1983). This may be a potential marker for sarcomas.

6

Special Tumors Occurring at Different Sites

ADAMANTINOMA OF THE TIBIA

Endothelium-related (factor VIII-related) antigen and epithelial (keratin) markers were investigated in an adamantinoma of the tibia (Rosai and Pinkus, 1982). The epithelial nature and not endothelial was established by the presence of keratin in tumor cells. Factor VIII-related antigen was present in endothelial cells only, not in tumor cells.

MESOTHELIOMAS

Mesothelial cells could be differentiated from adenocarcinoma cells in fluids on the basis of a 63,000 dalton keratin (Walts et al., 1984). It was detected in mesothelial cells, but not in adenocarcinomas, when tested by an immunoperoxidase technique. In addition mesothelioma cells in 49% of 37 patients contained hyaluronic acid, but the carcinoma cells of the 25 metastatic carcinoma cases examined did not (Kwee et al., 1982).

Pleural Mesotheliomas

Pleural mesotheliomas can be distinguished from pulmonary adenocarcinomas by the presence of keratin proteins and lack of CEA in the tumor cells (Corson and Pinkus, 1982). On the other hand, adenocarcinomas contained more CEA and very little or no keratin proteins. If the concentration of CEA in the pleural fluid exceeded 15 ng/ml the probability of the presence of a mesothelioma was zero (Faravelli et al., 1984).

Localized Fibrous Mesothelioma

Using keratins of different molecular weights as tumor markers, it was demonstrated immunohistochemically that localized fibrous mesotheliomas differed from mesotheliomas (Said et al., 1984). They did not contain keratins typically present in mesotheliomas. Ultrastructurally the tumor cells resembled mesenchymal cells. They probably originated from pleural fibroblasts.

ADENOMATOID TUMORS

These tumors are mesothelial derivatives. They contained immunohistochemically demonstrable keratin and no factor VIII (endothelial cell marker) or CEA (Said et al., 1982).

Another view is that these tumors constitute two groups: vascular and mesothelial (Bell and Flotte, 1982). It was possible to differentiate by the histochemical marker characteristics. The vascular adenomatoid tumors contained factor VIII-related antigen. The mesothelial adenomatoid tumors did not contain this antigen, but electron microscopically they resembled mesothelial cells.

GRANULAR CELL MYOBLASTOMAS

This tumor expresses a nonspecific cross-reacting antigen (NCA) that is related to CEA (Matthews and Mason, 1983). Histologically granular cell myoblastoma has characteristic cytoplasmic granulation observable with routine hematoxylin and eosin staining. Therefore NCA provides no contribution to histologic diagnosis.

CARCINOID TUMORS

The tumor-associated marker somatostatin is present predominantly in carcinoid tumors of foregut, of hindgut, and in intraintestinal sites (Dayal et al., 1982). This hormone is a useful histochemical marker for identifying carcinoids.

Another tumor-associated marker, neuron-specific enolase, was present in all 11 thymic carcinoids examined immunohistochemically (Wick et al., 1983).

S-100, a marker for neural crest-derived tumors, was present in carcinoid tumor cells (Ulich et al., 1982) also. These findings suggest that carcinoid tumors may be derived from the neural crest.

PHEOCHROMOCYTOMAS

Although endocrine hormone markers are well known and adequate for pheochromocytomas, it is possible to differentiate calcitonin-producing tumors from C-cell carcinomas by serum CEA determination (Cordes et al., 1983). While serum CEA is elevated in C-cell carcinomas, it is not increased in pheochromocytomas. All pheochromocytomas contained neuron-specific enolase, thus distinguishing medullary from cortical tumors (R.V. Lloyd et al., 1984). Cortical tumors and normal adrenal cortex gave negative immunohistochemical test results for this enolase.

MULTIPLE MYELOMAS

Microglobulin

Serum paraproteins are tumor markers to monitor the disease processes. In those cases where paraproteins are not produced, other markers can be measured.

Serum β_2-microglobulin was an indicator of prognosis (Child et al., 1983). It reflected the tumor burden. Serum levels before treatment correlated better than any other parameter with the survival of the patients. In addition, serum ferritin was a complementary marker to β_2-microglobulin (Linkesch and Ludwig, 1982).

A Myeloma-Associated Antigen

An antiserum to myeloma cells grown in tissue culture was raised in rabbits (Krueger et al., 1976). Using immunofluorescence microscopy, it was estimated that the appropriately absorbed antiserum reacted with myeloma cells and cells of benign monoclonal gammopathy in a significantly higher titer than with normal plasma cells.

Using an Ouchterlony immunodiffusion test, 25% of 16 patients had positive serum reactivity with another antiserum to lymphoma-associated antigen (LAA). This marker was highly specific for lymphomas and Hodgkin's disease (Udayachander et al., 1983).

There is evidence for a common antigen of IgG kappa (IgGK) myeloma cells (Hagner, 1983). Lymphocytes sensitized to autologous or allogeneic myeloma plasma cells lysed IgGK, but not IgG lambda cells.

By the use of a monoclonal antibody against human plasmacytoma cells it has been possible to differentiate normal and abnormal plasma cells from other lymphoid or myeloid cell types (Anderson et al., 1984). The antigen (PC-1) is shared by normal plasma cells from bone marrow and cells from plasma cell leukemias, plasmacytomas, and myelomas.

7

Malignant Lymphomas

NON-HODGKIN'S LYMPHOMAS (NHL)

In addition to morphologic recognition and classification, the NHL can be identified by tumor markers in patients' serum and cells. Many of the markers lack specificity for malignancy. However, they can be used to indicate the type of cells as to their origin. Some markers are highly specific for malignancy.

An oncofetal universal tumor marker, malignancy-associated nucleolar antigen (HMNA), is present in nucleoli of lymphoma cells only, not in the lymphocytes of hyperplastic lymph nodes, nor in activated lymphoid cells *in vitro* or growth-factor-dependent normal lymphoid cell lines (Ford, et al., 1984). The HMNA was detected using a heterologous antiserum to it. The HMNA was demonstrated in all 65 cases of T- and B-cell lymphomas.

Lymphoma-Associated Antigen (LAA)

A lymphoma-associated antigen (LAA) appeared as a tumor-specific marker (Udayachander et al., 1983). It was isolated from Hodgkin's and non-Hodgkin's lymph nodes and was found in the sera of lymphoma patients at concentrations of 152–830 ng/ml. LAA was not detected in sera from controls. This protein had an electrophoretic mobility at pH 8.6 as an α-globulin and a molecular weight of 29,600 by Sephadex G-200 chromatography and 43,000 by density/gradient centrifugation.

Modified Nucleosides

Modified nucleosides, especially psi, correlated with the clinical stages of malignant lymphomas including Hodgkin's disease (Rasmuson et al., 1982). In 4% of healthy adults, urine contained elevated levels of psi. In stage I, and in advanced disease, elevated urine levels occurred in 14% and 62% of patients, respectively.

Serum Deoxythymidine Kinase

Serum deoxythymidine kinase (S-dTK) levels correlated with the extent of disease and the aggressiveness of the tumor according to the Kiel histologic classification. S-dTK increased as the disease progressed and decreased following therapy in remission (Gronowitz et al., 1983). If the S-dTK level was high before treatment, patients with stage III or IV disease had a poor prognosis.

Serum Lactic Dehydrogenase (S-LDH)

Serum LDH was elevated in 41% of 113 patients with lymphomas (Endrizzi et al., 1982). Except for stage IV patients, normal values of LDH were associated with a better response to therapy and longer survival, regardless of the type and the clinical stage. In stages III and IV S-LDH reflected the spread of the disease and the histological grade of malignancy (Hagberg and Siegbahn, 1983). Of 155 untreated patients 80% survived a 2-year period when their S-LDH level was lower, while only 30% survived with high S-LDH. Besides this kind of prognostic value, S-LDH could be used to estimate the effect of therapy.

T-Cell Lymphomas

Among various subunits of T-cell lymphomas, there is one, cutaneous T-cell lymphoma, that can be identified by its relationship to HTLV.

HTLV

A type C retrovirus (HTLV) was isolated from blood and a lymph node of a patient with cutaneous T-cell lymphoma (mycosis fungoides), which is somewhat related to Hodgkin's disease (Reitz et al., 1981a). This appeared to be a new class of type C virus in man. A similar virus was isolated also from T-cell lymphoma-leukemia—Sézary's syndrome (Reitz et al., 1981b). This virus is evidently a characteristic human retrovirus and probably is closely associated with induction of these special T-cell lymphomas. It was demonstrated for the first time (Posner et al., 1981) that there were specific antibodies to a retrovirus in humans. These antibodies were directed against HTLV core proteins with molecular weights of 19,000 and 24,000. The specificity of this p24 protein was established by precipitation inhibition (Kalyanaraman et al., 1981). Antiserum to disrupted HTLV precipitated labeled p24. The precipitation was completed only by unlabeled HTLV and proteins from human cells producing HTLV.

There is a cluster of Japanese patients who have high titers of antibodies to HTLV in their serum (Robert-Guroff et al., 1982). It is possible that unique cell surface proteins defined by monoclonal antibodies to cutaneous T-cell lymphoma (Berger et al., 1981) have some relationship to HTLV activities.

In addition, Sézary's syndrome and mycosis fungoides share some functional properties in that they possess helper T-cell affinity to skin (Lawrence et al., 1978). The T-cell nature can be identified immunohistochemically in frozen sections by use of monoclonal antibodies to T-cells (Thomas and Janossy, 1982).

Besides the cutaneous lymphomas, which could be considered as a subset of the helper T-cell type, there is another group with suppressor T cells. The suppressor T cells can be differentiated from the helper T cells by the following characteristics: they are IgM-Fc receptor-negative, IgG-Fc receptor-positive, and acid nonspecific esterase-negative, and they contain azurophil granules. The helper T cell type has characteristics that are just the opposite of this pattern of markers (Stein et al., 1981). One monoclonal antibody to cutaneous T-cell lymphoma (CTCL) (BE1) precipitated an antigen with two components (Berger et al., 1982), which had molecular weights of 27,200 and 25,800. This and another monoclonal antibody to CTCL reacted with peripheral blood lymphocytes in 76% of 21 patients with CTCL. In these 16 patients CTCL was considered a skin lesion only.

B-Cell Lymphomas

Displacement of Immunoglobulin Gene

A specific marker for B-cell lymphomas is rearrangement of the immunoglobulin gene (Cleary et al., 1984). Using the Southern blot hybridization technique with specific probes for light- and heavy-chain immunoglobulin constant regions it was found that only B-cell lymphoma had rearrangement of the clonal immunoglobulin gene. The expression of κ or λ light-chain immunoglobulins correlated with the rearrangements of the corresponding genes. In the absence of any other markers, the immunoglobulin gene rearrangement is a specific marker in differential diagnosis for this malignancy.

The group consists of several subdivisions with different morphological features and degrees of malignancy.

Centroblastic Lymphoma

This type has been separated according to the Kiel classification based on cytologic morphology (Lennert, 1978). It is a highly malignant lymphoma. The cells contained histochemically demonstrable immunoglobulin (H. Stein et al., 1980). In the 60% of the cases with an absolute monotypic light-chain pattern, the μ and λ chains were predominant. The other B-cell lymphomas with lower-grade malignancy consist of monoclonal cells expressing κ or λ light chains and μ heavy chains. Some patients have Waldenström's macroglobulinemia or IgM paraproteinemia.

A Subset of B-Cell Lymphomas

A monoclonal antibody (Ab89) to B-cell poorly differentiated lymphocytic lymphoma (D-PDL) reacted only with autologous lymphoma cells and 10% of B-cell D-PDL as well as B-cell chronic lymphocytic leukemia (Nadler et al., 1980). This apparently is a special subset of the lymphoma-leukemia group with a common specific antigen.

Epstein-Barr Virus

Several types of non-Hodgkin's lymphomas reacted with antibodies to Epstein-Barr virus-associated antigens (Lindemalm et al., 1983). Elevated titers to early antigen of the diffuse type was observed quite frequently. The prognosis was poor when antibodies to this antigen approached a titer of 1:20.

HODGKIN'S DISEASE

Oncofetal Markers

There are two such antigens, one with a slower electrophoretic mobility-(S) and one a faster-moving entity (F) (Order et al., 1974). Using immunoelectrophoresis method, F antigen was demonstrated in Hodgkin's disease tumor extracts and extracts of fetal liver, spleen, and thymus. S antigen appeared in Hodgkin's tumors, reticulum cell sarcomas, and lymphocytic thymomas. It was related to T cells.

Tumor-Associated Markers

Ferritin

Tumor-associated marker ferritin is elevated in the serum of patients with Hodgkin's disease (Dörn et al., 1983). Normal values ranged in women from 30 to 150 ng/ml and in men from 30 to 400 ng/ml. The highest values were observed in stages III and IV, with arithmetic means of 378 and 831 ng/ml, respectively. Serum ferritin levels decreased during remission and increased during progression of the disease. As in the patients with non-Hodgkin's lymphomas, there was elevation of basic (liver) ferritin in the serum of patients with disseminated disease and the patients had poor prognosis. Since this type of ferritin, as determined with radioimmunoassay using monospecific antibodies, is synthesized by reticuloendothelial cells, elevated serum levels may be due to a nonspecific reaction of these cells. The acidic (HeLa) type of ferritin was elevated in 94% of all untreated patients. It reflected the effect of therapy (Cazzola et al., 1983). This type of ferritin probably originates from tumor cells of various kinds as they are present in Hodgkin's lymphoma.

Lymphoma-Associated Antigen (LAA)

Lymphoma-associated antigen (LAA) is present also in the sera of patients with Hodgkin's disease (Udayachander et al., 1983). In all 12 cases examined the serum LAA levels ranged from 187 to 1,508 ng/ml, while it was not detectable in the controls.

Tumor-Specific Markers

It was suggested that an antigen appearing in cultured cells from Hodgkin's disease tumors might contain a neoantigen (Long et al., 1977). Some evidence was also presented (Favre et al., 1978) that a cell surface antigen could be a tumor-specific antigen.

A highly specific monoclonal antiserum (Ki-1) to Hodgkin's (H cells) and Sternberg-Reed cells (SR cells) reacted also with a small subset of normal lymphoid cells (Schwab et al., 1982). Nevertheless, it could be used to differentiate Hodgkin's lymphoma cells from other normal cells even if the latter contained the respective antigen. These normal cells could be recognized by their distinctly normal morphologic appearance.

There were unique nuclear DNA sequences in the cells of Hodgkin's lymphoma (Kufe et al., 1973a).

BURKITT'S LYMPHOMA

Specific Markers

Two unique proteins with a molecular weight of approximately 40,000 were present in the sera of 86% of patients with this disease and 80% of patients with nasopharyngeal carcinoma (Gazitt et al., 1981).

One of the major glycoprotein antigens (GP40) of the immune complexes in the sera of patients with Burkitt's lymphoma reacts with the antibodies from the sera of patients with different malignant neoplasms including colon carcinomas (Gazitt et al., 1983).

A glycolipid was identified using a monoclonal antibody directed to a Burkitt's lymphoma cell line (Nudelman et al., 1983). It was globotriaosylceramide [Galα(1$\rightarrow$4)Galβ(1$\rightarrow$4)Glcβ(1$\rightarrow$1)-ceramide]. Burkitt's lymphoma cells contained 100 times more of this glycolipid than did other leukemia or lymphoma cell lines.

Virus-Related Markers

Incorporation of the Epstein-Barr virus genome in some Burkitt's lymphomas is well-known. There are unique nuclear DNA sequences in the cells of Burkitt's lymphoma that cross-hybridized with those of Hodgkin's lymphoma cells (Kufe et al., 1973a). They were not related to the DNA of Epstein-Barr virus. In 13 of 15 patients, lymphoma cells contained particles with RNA-instructed DNA polymerase (Kufe et al., 1973b). There apparently was RNA homologous to RNA of Rauscher leukemia virus.

Oncogenes

C-*myc* oncogene product was expressed in large amounts as a result of specific chromosome translocations of light-chain loci from bands 2p11 and 22q11 to the 3′ region of the c-*myc* oncogene (Croce, 1984). However, the transforming gene *Blym 1* located on the short arm of chromosome Ip32 was not physically linked to the c-*myc* oncogene (Morton et al., 1984).

8

Leukemias

ONCOFETAL MARKERS

Human leukemic cell line K 562, isolated from a patient at blast crisis of chronic myelogenous leukemia, expressed a fetal-type cell surface antigen i (Fukuda, 1980a). When such a cell line was used to raise an immune serum in a rabbit, this antiserum induced a complement-mediated cytotoxicity of cells from myelogenous and lymphocytic leukemias (Whitson et al., 1976). The cytotoxicity titer was reduced by absorbing the immune serum with first-trimester human whole-embryo cells. An immune serum raised in rabbits with cells of acute myeloblastic leukemia cross-reacted also with the sera of patients with acute and chronic lymphocytic and myelogenous leukemias and some patients with Hodgkin disease, and with fetal serum (Harris et al., 1971).

Apparently, there are antigenic similarities among fetal liver, the cells of acute lymphocytic leukemia, and lymphosarcoma (Thränhardt et al., 1978). An antiserum to fetal liver reacted in *in vitro* cytotoxic tests with these cells. There was no reaction with the cells of acute myelogenous leukemia or chronic lymphocytic leukemia. However, an antigen (LAA) with the characteristics of α_2-β-globulin present in fetal liver and amniotic fluid was present also in the sera of patients with acute and chronic myelogenous leukemia as well as in some healthy individuals (Berg et al., 1977).

There is an oncofetal antigen that cross-reacts among human and mice fetal liver and acute lymphocytic and myelogenous leukemias (Granatek et al., 1976).

Fetal tissues other than liver contain an antigen that cross-reacts with leukemia. An antiserum was raised with fetal tissues of 10 weeks gestation after the removal of brain, spinal cord, and viscera. This antiserum cross-reacted with an antigen on the plasma membranes of cultured B-cell lines but not with a cultured T-cell line or with thymocytes (Sullivan et al., 1976). This antigen was prominent and in higher percentages of cells of chronic lymphocytic leukemia. A significantly smaller percentage of normal peripheral blood lymphocytes reacted with the fetal antiserum.

Of all the above-mentioned markers the most useful at this time may be the human malignancy-associated nucleolar antigen (HMNA). The percentage of bone marrow cells with the presence of HMNA was 9% to 98% with a median of 83% in all 72 patients with acute leukemia (Davis et al., 1984). In nonleukemic individuals the range was 0.05% to 2.5% with a median of 1%. In remission patients had a significant decrease of HMNA-positive cells varying from 0 to 83% with a median of 3%. Some of the blast cells were HMNA-negative and some partially differentiated ones were HMNA-positive. As the patients approached a relapse, the number of HMNA-positive cells increased.

TUMOR-ASSOCIATED MARKERS

An antigen (HThy-L) of molecular weight 40,000–50,000 was isolated from human thymocytes. A component of this HThy-L antigen with a molecular weight of 43,000 possessed an antigenic activity also in cultured T-cell lines and red blood cell rosette-positive leukemia blast cells (Chechik et al., 1978a). Using radioimmunoassay Chechik et al. (1979) found significant quantitative differences among different cells. The highest HThy-L concentration was in the normal thymocytes, T-cell lines, and red blood cell rosette-positive acute lymphoblastic leukemia cells. A thymus-leukemia-associated antigen was identified on leukemic T-cell lines and normal thymocytes (Seon et al., 1980). The largest component of this antigen had a molecular weight of approximately 68,000. Serum ferritin levels reflected probability of survival of patients under 60 years of age (Ogier et al., 1984).

Multiple Enzyme Markers in Acute Leukemias

The various enzyme patterns related to acute leukemias according to the French-American-British classification are indicated in Table 1 (condensed from Table 2 of Drexler et al., 1984).

The typical enzyme pattern for any recorded leukemia serves to differentiate it from the rest of this group. On the basis of these enzyme markers it is not possible to differentiate AMMoL from AMoL. Acute undifferentiated leukemia in spite of the presence of various enzyme markers (Drexler et al., 1984) could not be differentiated from the ALL, cALL, Null-ALL, B-ALL, and Non-T/Non-B-ALL.

Terminal Deoxynucleotidyl Transferase (TdT) in Leukemias

This enzyme is present in varying amounts in different leukemic cells. It was found to be a useful marker for identification of acute lymphoblastic

Table 1. Enzyme Patterns Related to Acute Leukemia (according to French-American-British classification)

Type of leukemia	Markers						
	5′-Nucleotidase (5′-N)	Purine-nucleoside phosphorylase (PNP)	Terminal transferase (TdT)	Alkaline phosphatase (AP)	Cytidine deaminase	α-D-Galactosidase	Lysozyme
Acute lymphoblastic (ALL)					Normal		Normal or decreased
Acute myeloblastic (AML)					Decreased		
Common acute lymphoblastic (CALL)	Increased						
Null acute lymphoblastic (Null-ALL)	Normal	Decreased					
B-cell acute lymphoblastic (B-ALL)			Normal				
T-cell acute lymphoblastic (T-ALL)						Decreased	
Non-T/Non-B Acute lymphoblastic (Non-T/Non-B-ALL)				Increased			
Acute myelomonoblastic (AMMoL)						Increased	Increased
Acute monoblastic (AMoL)						Increased	Increased

leukemias (Srivastava et al., 1980). High TdT activity was present also in acute myelocytic cells, but not as frequently as in acute lymphoblastic leukemias. Using immunofluorescence microscopy (Froelich et al., 1981), it was possible to demonstrate TdT on normal cells. The number of TdT-positive cells correlated with the clinical course. When the number of TdT-positive cells increased more than 0.1% of the peripheral mononuclear cells, there was an imminent relapse, while during remission the number of such cells remained less than 0.1%. In T-cell acute lymphoblastic leukemia lacking Ia antigens (Bradstock et al., 1981) the presence of TdT-positive cells in bone marrow specifically indicated early relapse or the presence of residual disease.

This enzyme alone cannot provide complete information in differential diagnosis. Within a context of "multiple marker analysis" (Drexler et al., 1984) it is a helpful marker.

Histiocytic Esterase in Leukemias

It is possible to differentiate histiocytic-monocytic leukemias, as well as lymphomas, from other such proliferative lymphopathies on the basis of ultrastructural cytochemical techniques demonstrating histiocytic esterase with 2-naphthyl thiol acetate as the substrate (Kim et al., 1982).

LEUKEMIA-SPECIFIC MARKERS

There are now a great number of marker antigens for leukemias that facilitate the recognition of different variants of the disease (Metzgar and Mohanakumar, 1977). These antigens are not yet defined, although evidence for the existence of leukemia-specific gene products has been presented earlier (Viza et al., 1970). Using heterologous antisera to leukemic cells (Pollack et al., 1977) or autologous and allogeneic immune sera (Nadkarin et al., 1973), determination of specific antigen was applied to clinical evaluation of the leukemic diseases. An antiserum in a monkey was raised with a surface glycoprotein from cells of a patient with acute myeloblastic leukemia (Mohanakumar et al., 1981). This antiserum reacted specifically with different leukemias. There is also evidence (Iqbal and Rothenberg, 1981) that nonfunctional dihydrofolate reductase of human leukemia cells shares antigenic determinants with a functional form of that enzyme from LI210 mouse leukemia cells.

Many attempts have been made to detect specific tumor markers for different kinds of leukemias, lymphocytic and myelogenous, acute, and chronic as well as antigens or compounds related to viruses. A monoclonal antibody raised to the common acute lymphoblastic leukemia cell line Reh reacted exclusively with 69% of non-B, non-T ALL, 50% of T-ALL, 18% of AML, and 66% of CML blast crisis cells (Billing et al., 1982). Other different cell types did not react with this antibody. The antigen appeared to be a blast cell antigen.

Antigens Cross-reacting With RAJI Cells

A rabbit antiserum to the RAJI cell line derived from a patient with Burkitt lymphoma was cytotoxic to cells of acute myelocytic or lymphocytic leukemias (Mann et al., 1974). This antigen appeared in the acute phase of the disease and disappeared in the remission. The relationship to viruses can be suggested by the observations that this antigen is not expressed by embryonic kidney cells, but appears after infection with Rauscher, Kirsten, or SV40 viruses. It may be that the leukemia-specific antisera (Billing and Terasaki, 1974; Pandolfi et al., 1977) reacting with RAJI cells contained antibodies to this antigen. There were antibodies in the sera of patients with hairy cell leukemia (Cassareale et al., 1981) cross-reacting with Epstein-Barr virus-related antigens.

ACUTE MYELOBLASTIC LEUKEMIAS

Calcitonin

Serum calcitonin levels exceeded 1,000 pg/ml in 45% of the patients with acute leukemia and in blast crisis with chronic myelocytic leukemia (Pflüger et al., 1982).Remissions and relapses were reflected in the serum calcitonin levels. Such an elevation of calcitonin was not observed in chronic leukemias and in lymphomas. Furthermore, besides the physiological calcitonin the serum of these patients with elevated levels contained high-molecular-weight forms. Only such entities were present in the leukemic cells, indicating that they are the source of the serum hormone.

Pterins

6-Hydroxmethylpterin levels in urine accurately reflected the remission of the disease by a decrease in concentration (Trehan et al., 1982). This marker correlated also with the percentage of blasts and thus indicted the status of the disease.

Specific Antigens in Acute Myeloblastic Leukemias

It is possible that a glycoprotein with a molecular weight of 350,000–400,000 represents a unique marker for myoblastic leukemia cells (Taub et al., 1978). Antisera to HLA or B-cell antigens did not react to this antigen. There is also strong evidence for a specific antigen in the blast cells of myelogenous leukemia (Al-Rammahy et al., 1980). An immune serum to acute myelogenous leukemia cells reacted specifically with blast cells from leukemia patients, not with normal bone marrow cells. Specific antisera to human leukemic blast cells have been produced in mice that are tolerant to remission leukocytes from the same individual (Baker et al., 1974). There is a possibility that a coarsely granular nuclear antigen in leukemia lymphoblasts is a tumor-specific entity (Klein et al., 1974).

A human-human hybridoma antibody (am1-18) reacted specifically with mononuclear peripheral cells of 41% of 54 acute myeloblastic leukemia cases (Olsson et al., 1984). There was no correlation between the pattern of reactivity and the types of leukemia. In addition, 2 of 4 samples from patients with acute lymphoblastic leukemia reacted with this antibody also.

PROMYELOCYTIC LEUKEMIAS

A specific marker has been detected for promyelocytic leukemias (Aota et al., 1982). It is a monoclonal antibody (WI-1) raised against a promyelocytic cell line, H2-60. The antibody reacts with an antigen with a molecular weight of 42,000.

CHRONIC MYELOGENOUS LEUKEMIAS

Lipid-Associated Sialic Acid (LSA)

Lipid-associated sialic acid (LSA), a universal tumor-associated marker is present in the serum at levels above 20 mg% in 85% of patients with chronic myelogenous leukemia (Katopodis et al., 1983). The sensitivity of this marker can be improved by analyzing the serum sample immediately. Delay causes a decrease of LSA at a rate of 1% per hour.

An Antigen in Neoplastic Granulocytes

This antigen is a glycoprotein and served as a marker for neoplastic granulocytes when used with the immunoperoxidase microscopy technique (Pattengale et al., 1980). It was helpful in identifying primitive cells originating from granulocytic series. This antigen was present also on normal granulocytes, but not on normal lymphoid cells. Similarly, an antigen specific for myeloid leukemia and normal cells reacted with an antiserum raised in rabbits with purified membrane extracts of myelogenous leukemia cells (Malcolm et al., 1982).

ACUTE LYMPHOBLASTIC LEUKEMIA (ALL)

Modified Nucleosides

Modified nucleosides were significantly elevated in urine in childhood ALL (Heldman et al., 1983). They served as markers of the activity of the disease. Among N_2N_2-dimethylguanosine, 1-methylguanosine, pseudouridine, and 1-methylinosine the latter correlated the best with the percentage of blast cells in the bone marrow.

Specific Antigens in Acute Lymphoblastic Leukemias (ALL)

Among a variety of glycoproteins with a molecular weight of approximately 100,000, there are some tumor-specific antigens. At least one such antigen was detected by use of a common acute lymphoblastic leukemia antiserum (Pesando et al., 1980). Extensively absorbing a rabbit immune serum to ALL cells, it was possible to isolate such a specific antigen (Kabisch et al., 1978). It yielded two chromatographically separate entities with molecular weights of approximately 55,000 and 110,000. From another study, ALL-specific antigen appeared to have a molecular weight in the same range—98,000 (Billing et al., 1978).

Common acute lymphoblastic leukemia antigens (CALLA) have been used in identification of different patterns of leukemia (Brown et al., 1979). This antigen reacted with non-T-, non-B-cell acute lymphoblastic leukemias, T-cell leukemias, and B-cell lymphomas (Minowada et al., 1978). Using monoclonal antibodies to CALLA, it was found in common and late thymocytes (Barnard et al., 1981); therefore, some of its components may not be specific for malignant lymphoid cells.

A specific antigen in ALL is suspected from studies with an antibody in a serum of a patient with ALL (Naito et al., 1983). It reacted in immunoadherence assays with autologous leukemia cells, but not with the cells in remission. This reactivity was inhibited by adsorption of serum with ALL cells from 10 of 14 patients. No other cell lines, including those expressed by HTLV reacted with inhibition of the reaction.

It appeared that there is a tumor-specific antigen in the T-cell-type acute lymphoblastic leukemia (T-ALL). The monospecific antibody SN1 raised against a leukemia antigen from a T-ALL cell line did not react with any other cell type, benign or malignant, except those of T-ALL (Seon et al., 1983). This unique antigen was designated TALLA. The molecular weight of a unique T-ALL antigen was 100,000 (Mohanakumar et al., 1983). It was a membrane component of T-ALL.

CHRONIC LYMPHOCYTIC LEUKEMIAS

BLA antigen expression was studied with a monoclonal antibody 38.13 (Klein et al., 1983). BLA was expressed strongly by chronic lymphocytic leukemia cells and B-cell lymphomas. Three centroblastic lymphomas examined were negative for BLA, while immunocytomas were reacting weakly. Thus it appeared that the expression of BLA was related to the degree of differentiation.

B-Cell Type

It is suggested that a gene designated as *bcl-1* (B-cell lymphoma/leukemia), located on the 14q+ chromosome, becomes activated by this translocation in chronic lymphocytic leukemia and large-cell lymphoma cells (Tsujimoto et al., 1984). Furthermore, it was suggested that the *bcl-1* gene is not homologous to any of the known retroviral oncogenes. This was t(11:14) translocation. Normally chromosome 11 contained the *bcl-1* locus. The product of this translocation may be a marker for some of these leukemias and lymphomas.

HAIRY CELL LEUKEMIA

Three monoclonal antibodies reacted with hairy cells with a high degree of specificity (Posnett et al., 1982). One of them was most specific, reacting only with hairy cells but not with the cells of all patients. The other antibodies that reacted with 100% sensitivity reacted also with some other cell types.

A unique membrane protein, p35, has been demonstrated in hairy cells of both Japanese and white patients (Katayama et al., 1984). Further differentiation of hairy cell leukemia from other B-cell types may be possible by use of a monoclonal antibody (Posnett et al., 1984). This antibody (αHCl) was raised against hairy cell leukemia cells. It did not react with other B-cell types or normal cells but cross-reacted with epithelial basal cells and endothelial cells except those in brain and sinusoids of spleen and liver.

VIRUSES

There have been numerous studies in search for viruses in human leukemias. In 24 of 27 leukemia patients studied, there was RNA in the leukemia cells that was homologous to RNA of the Rauscher leukemia virus (Hehlmann et al., 1972). It was not present in normal adult or fetal tissues, but was found in human sarcomas. Human leukemia cells contained an RNA homologous to the RNA of woolly monkey sarcoma viruses (Gallo, 1976).

Also, group and specific antigens of woolly monkey sarcoma virus and gibbon ape leukemia virus were present in human leukemia cells. The RNA-directed DNA transcriptase activity in human cells was inhibited by antibodies to such an enzyme of the primate RNA viruses. There is also evidence (Metzgar et al., 1976) that cells of human chronic granulocytic and acute myelogenous leukemia share membrane antigens with p30 and gp71 of the Friend murine leukemia virus.

In white blood cells or plasma of patients with leukemias, there was evidence of antigens cross-reacting with p28 antigen of baboon endogenous virus, p30 of simian sarcoma virus, gp70 of Rauscher mouse leukemia virus, and gp70 of gibbon ape leukemia virus (Vaczi and Toth, 1980). In one family member with familial acute myelogenous leukemia, serum RNA-directed DNA polymerase activity was elevated (Sadamori et al., 1981). A high proportion of mononuclear cells of acute leukemia contained antigens cross-reacting with antisera of nonhuman primate C-type viruses or their major internal proteins (Pullen and Hersey, 1981). There is now evidence that antigens of 36% of 86 leukemia patients cross-reacted with antibodies to p30 of Simian sarcoma-associated virus (SiSV) and antigens of 40% of 48 patients cross-reacted with antibodies to p30 of baboon endogenous viruses (BaEV) (Hehlmann et al., 1983). The leukemias included acute myelomonocytic, acute myeloblastic, acute promyelocytic, acute lymphoblastic, chronic myelogenous, and blast crisis. There was a common human antigen with a molecular weight of 70,000. The major peptides of human antigens had identical mobilities with 11 of 21 major peptides of SiSV p30 and 10 of 20 peptides of BaEV p30. These markers were specific and could be of diagnostic and prognostic significance. The significance of the expression of these antigens is not known.

Human T-Cell Leukemia Virus (HTLV)

A human type C RNA tumor virus (HTLV) was isolated from patients with T-cell leukemias and lymphomas (Gallo and Wong-Staal, 1982). Its core protein p24 is evolutionarily related to p24 of bovine leukemia virus. While a few cases with antibodies to HTLV have been detected in the USA, there is an endemic area with adult T-cell leukemias and T-cell lymphomas in southwestern Japan and Caribbean West Indies populations. In those endemic areas, not only the patients, but also apparently healthy individuals had a high frequency of antibodies to HTLV. Some people whose sera are negative for antibodies may still be infected by the HTLV (Sarin et al., 1983). A brother of a patient with HTLV had serum negative for HTLV, but his T-cell line expressed p19, p24, and reverse transcriptase with type C virus particles. On the other hand, a patient's mother had a positive serum reaction for HTLV, and abnormal peripheral blood lymphocytes with expression of HTLV antigens, but no clinical evidence of the disease. HTLV p19 can serve as a marker for the diagnosis of viral infection. It was located on the cell surface and viruses (Aoki et al., 1984). A monoclonal antibody (IgG1) to p19 did not induce cytotoxicity or lyse cells in the presence of complement.

The mode of infection by HTLV and the frequency of the resulting disease is not yet known. In addition, a subtype of this HTLV virus was also demonstrated. It differed from the HTLV-I in the immunological reactivities testing p24 the internal core protein (Kalyanaraman et al., 1982). This subtype was designated HTLV-II. It was isolated from a case of hairy cell leukemia. To the group of HTLV belongs a virus that is associated with the acquired immune deficiency syndrome (Gallo et al., 1983). Four types of monoclonal antibodies to p24 have been developed (Palker et al., 1984) and can be used as diagnostic reagents to identify HTLV- and HTLV-II-infected cells.

Adult T-Cell Leukemia Virus (ATLV)

Adult T-cell leukemia (ATL) is associated with a retrovirus (ATLV) that was demonstrated in a cell line from a patient with ATL (Hinuma, 1983). The ATLV relationship to HTLV is not know, but it is possible that they are the same species (Gallo and Reitz, 1982).

The ATLV antigen (ATLA) contains a glycoprotein (gp46) with a molecular weight of 46,000 that may constitute the viral envelope glycoprotein (Yamamoto, 1983). ATLV induces ATLA in normal human T as well as B cells by infecting them. Using indirect immunoelectron microscopy it was observed (Nakai, 1983) that some human sera containing antibodies to ATLA reacted with ATLV particles and the surface of the MT-2 cell membranes. Thus it was suggested that ATLA is a marker for this type C particle, the ATLV.

Antibodies to ATLA were detected in 29% of 82 patients with T-cell malignancies (Tobinani et al., 1983), but not in 106 patients with B-cell malignancies. Among the T-cell malignancies there were the highest incidences of antibodies to ATLA (45% of 51 patients) in OKT4-positive mature T-cell (inducer/helper T-cell) malignancies. In a case of T-cell derived chronic lymphocytic leukemia ATLA was detected in the cells after a short-term culture (Utsunomiya et al., 1983). The patient had antibodies to ATLA.

At least 5 cases of adult T-cell leukemia-lymphoma have been studied and no antibodies were detected to adult T-cell leukemia virus antigen (Shimoyama et al., 1983). In one case antibody was expressed after the culturing of the leukemia cells. In other cases there was no expression of such antibodies after a long-term culturing of the cells. It is possible that in this group of patients, if the leukemia was induced by the human leukemia virus, there was no immunological response. Another alternative is the possibility of a T-cell leukemia entity without the viral involvement.

Cells expressing ATLV contained gp68, a possible precursor of viral envelope polypeptides (Schneider et al., 1984). Viral particles contained p24, p19, p15, and small amounts of gp46, which appeared to be loosely attached to the viral and cell surfaces. The ATL antigen complex appeared to contain viral structural proteins.

ATLV binds specifically not only to T cells, but to various other hematopoietic cells, including B, non-T, and non-B lines (Yamamoto et al., 1984).

Antibodies to ATLV-associated antigens were also present in Japanese and imported monkeys (Hayami et al., 1984). The incidence of the presence of the antigen increased with the age of the animals, a relation similar to findings from observations of human subjects. The direct transmission from animals to humans appeared unlikely owing to distinct differences of the geographical distribution of the monkeys and the human subjects. It was demonstrated (Gotoh et al., 1982) that healthy people carry ATLV in their circulatory T lymphocytes.

ONCOGENES IN LEUKEMIAS

DNA sequences related to the c-*myc* gene have been amplified in a human myeloid leukemia cell line (Collins and Groudine, 1982), and amplification of c-*abl* with concomitant amplification of sequences for an immunoglobulin light-chain constant region was present in a CML cell line (Heisterkamp et al., 1983).

In the cell lines of a patient with acute myelogenous leukemia, there was a fivefold to tenfold amplification of the c-*myb* oncogene (Pelicci et al., 1984) with a corresponding high level of transcription. These cell lines had karyotypic rearrangements associated with chromosome 6, the normal site of the c-*myb* locus.

An 8.2-kb c-*abl*-related mRNA was present in three cell lines of Philadelphia chromosome-positive chronic myelogenous leukemia cell lines and in a fresh leukemia cell sample (Collins et al., 1984). The *abl*-related mRNA was not present in nonleukemic cell lines. This mRNA was up to 8 times higher in the cell lines from the stages of blast crisis than in cells during chronic phase or in nonleukemia cells. Oncogene c-*abl* is translocated from band 34 of chromosome 9 to band 11 of chromosome 22. This translocation is accompanied by a translocation of c-*sis* from chromosome 22 to 9 (Bartram et al., 1984).

IMMUNOTHERAPY

With the availability of monoclonal antibodies that would bind to specific antigens in tumor cells only, attempts have been made to apply immunotherapy. Use of heterologous monoclonal antibodies, however, induces undesirable side effects. With small doses of antibody such reactions can be avoided (Foon et al., 1983). There was about a 50% reduction of the circulating cell counts in some of the CLL patients treated with a monoclonal antibody to a 65,000 molecular weight antigen (T65).

Conclusions

Tumor-associated markers representing various normal adult gene products have been well defined and their use in clinical medicine well established.

Oncofetal tumor markers for human malignant neoplasms, with the exception of HCG, have been studied for only the past 15 years. Two of them, CEA and AFP, have found wide clinical application. TPA may be a marker with a potential similar to that of CEA. There are, however, several isoproteins of these markers that have not yet been precisely defined.

The least-known of the three types of markers are tumor-specific products. While there is clear evidence of tumor-specific transplantation antigens in animal malignant neoplasms, specifically mutated oncogenes, such entities have not been well documented or well defined in patients. It is in this area that further studies of both universal tumor-specific markers and those with more limited specificity may reveal their nature—tumor-specific, tumor-associated, or oncofetal. Once such markers are detected, immunodiagnosis and therapy will be more effective than the present attempts using markers with limited specificity.

References

Abad EA, Lluch G Jr (1980): C_1 esterase inhibitor protein associated with human cancer: A tumor marker. Rev Esp Oncol 27:563–569.

Ablin RJ, Gonder MJ, Soanes WA (1974): Immunohistological studies of carcinoma of the prostate. III. Elution of interepithelial antibodies from carcinomatous human prostatic tissue following cryoprostatectomy. Oncology 29:329–334.

Adelusi B (1982): Tumour-associated antigens in cervical cancer tissues and in the sera of Nigerian women with cervical cancer. Afr J Med Med Sci 11:123–127.

Agashe SS, Gangal SG, Nair PNM, Rao RS (1977): Blocking of oncofetal cross-reactivity in human osteogenic sarcoma with solubilized tumour antigen. Indian J Med Res 66:824–831.

Alitalo K, Schwab M, Lin CC, Varmus HE, Bishop JM (1983): Homogeneously staining chromosomal regions contain amplified copies of an abundantly expressed cellular oncogene (c-myc) in malignant neuroendocrine cells from a human colon carcinoma. Proc Natl Acad Sci USA 80:1707–1711.

Allerton S, Powars D, Beierle J, Chen C, Wise K (1976): Wilms' tumor: Associated proteoglycans and glycoprotein antigen. Proc Am Soc Clin Oncol 17:292.

Al-Rammahy AK, Shipman S, Jackson A, Malcolm A, Levy, JG (1981): Evidence for a common leukemia-associated antigen in acute myelogenous leukemia. Cancer Immunol Immunother 9:181–185.

Andersen MM (1979): Studies of ferritin in renal carcinoma. Protides Biol Fluid Proc Colloq 27:347–350.

Anderson KC, Bates MP, Slaughenhoupt B, Schlossman SF, Nadler LM (1984): A monoclonal antibody with reactivity restricted to normal and neoplastic plasma cells. J Immunol 132:3172–3179.

Aoki N, DeGroot LJ (1982): Inhibition of leukocyte migration by human thyroid adenocarcinoma associated antigens. Acta Endocrinol (Copenh) 99:56–63.

Aoki T, Hamada C, Ohno S, Miyakoshi H, Konde H, Robert-Guroff M, Ting RC, Gallo RC (1984): Location of human T-cell leukemia virus (HTLV) p19 antigen on virus-producing cells. Int J Cancer 33:161–165.

Aota F, Chang D, Hill NO, Khan A (1982): Monoclonal antibody against a unique antigen on human acute promyelocytic leukemia cell line (HL-60). Exp Hematol 10:835–843.

Ariyoshi Y, Kato K, Ishiguro Y, Ota K, Sato T, Suchi T (1983a): Evaluation of serum neuron-specific enolase as a tumor marker for carcinoma of the lung. Gann 74:219–225.

Ariyoshi Y, Kato K, Ishiguro Y, Ota K, Sato T, Suchi T (1983b): Marker-specific enolase as a new tumor marker. Gan To Kagaku Ryoho 10:1744–1453.

Arnold W, Klein M, Wang JB, Schmidt WAK, Trampisch HJ (1981): Coronavirus-associated antibodies in nasopharyngeal carcinoma and infectious mononucleosis. Arch Otorhinolaryngol 232:165–177.

Aron M, Egly JM, Isaac JP (1974): Recherches serologiques, immunologiques et immunochimiques sur la presence d'une proteine antigene specifique dans l'urine des canceraux. Arch Anat Histol Embryol 56:165–179.

Arya SK, Zeigel RF, Horoszewicz JS, Carter WA (1976): RNA tumor virus-like activities in human solid tissues: Endogenous RNA:DNA polymerase activities in the prostate. J Surg Oncol 8:321–332.

Asaka M, Nagase K, Miyazaki T, Alpert E (1983): Aldolase A isoenzyme levels in serum and tissues of patients with liver disease. Gastroenterology 84:155–160.

Ashall F, Bramwell ME, Harris H (1982): A new marker for human cancer cells. I. The Ca antigen and the Cal antibody. Lancet 2:1–6.

Aurelian L, Kessler II, Rosenshein NB, Barbour G (1981): Viruses and gynecologic cancers: Herpesvirus protein (ICP 10/AG-4) a cervical tumor antigen that fulfills the criteria for a marker of carcinogeneity. Cancer 48:455–471.

Awais GM (1983): Dysgerminoma and serum lactic dehydroginase levels. Obstet Gynecol 61:99–101.

Axel R, Schlom J, Spiegelman S (1972a): Presence in human breast cancer of RNA homologous to mouse mammary tumour virus RNA. Nature 235:32–36.

Axel R, Gulati SC, Spiegelman S (1972b): Particles containing RNA-instructed DNA polymerase and virus-related RNA in human breast cancers. Proc Natl Acad Sci USA 69:3133–3137.

Azzarone B, Suarez H, Mingari M-C, Moretta L, Fauci AS (1984): 4F2 monoclonal antibody recognizes a surface antigen on spread human fibroblasts of embryonic but not of adult origin. J Cell Biol 98:1133–1137.

Babian RJ, Swanson DA (1982): Serum haptoglobin: A nonspecific tumor marker for renal cell carcinoma. South Med J 75:1345–1348.

Baker LH, Mebusz WK, Chin TD, Chapman AL, Hinthorn D, Towle D (1981): The relationship of herpesvirus to carcinoma of the prostate. J Urol 125:370–374.

Baker MA, Ramachandar K, Taub RN (1974): Specificity of heteroantisera to human acute leukemia-associated antigens. J Clin Invest 54:1273–1278.

Bakowski MT, Toseland PA, Wicks JF, Trounce JR (1981): A rapid gas chromatographic method for the determination of plasma polyamines and its application to the prediction of tumour response to chemotherapy. Clin Chim Acta 110:273–286.

Balis ME, Higgins PJ, Salser JS (1981): Enzymes of normal, premalignant, and malignant colonic cells. In Bruce WR, Correa P, Lipkin M, Tannenbaum SR, Wilkins TD (eds): "Banbury Report 7, Gastrointestinal Cancer: Endogenous Factors." Cold Spring Harbor Laboratory, NY: Cold Spring Harbor Laboratory, pp 129–139.

Banwo O, Versey J, Hobbs JR (1974): New oncofetal antigen for human pancreas. Lancet 1:643–645.

Bara J, Paul-Gardais A, Loisillier F, Burtin P (1978): Isolation of a sulfated glycopeptidic antigen from human gastric tumors: Its localization in normal and cancerous gastrointestinal tissues. Int J Cancer 21:133–139.

Barbolin VI, Gabuniia AI, Abramov VF (1980): Carcinoembryonic antigen in evaluating the efficacy of treatment of lung cancer patients. USSR Med Radiol (Mosk) 25:12–16.

Barnard A, Boumsell L, Reinherz EL, Nadler LM, Ritz J, Coppin H, Richard Y, Valensi F, Dausset J, Flandrin G, Lemerle J, Schlossman SF (1981): Cell surface characterization of malignant T cells from lymphoblastic lymphoma using monoclonal antibodies: Evidence for phenotypic differences between malignant T cells from patients with acute lymphoblastic leukemia and lymphoblastic lymphoma. Blood 57:1105–1110.

Bartram CR, DeKlein A, Hagemeijer A, Grosveld G, Heisterkamp N, Groffen J (1984): Localization of the human c-sis oncogene in Ph′-positive and Ph′-negative chronic myelocytic leukemia by in situ hybridization. Blood 63:223–225.

Bashford J, Gough IR (1983): Depression of high-affinity rosette formation in dysplasia and carcinoma in situ of the uterine cervix: Mediation by serum factors. Cancer Res 43:3959–3962.

Bast RC, Klug T, St. John ES, Jenison E, Niloff J, Lazarus J, Derkowitz R, Leavitt T, Griffiths CT, Parker L, Zurawski V, Knapp RC (1983): A radioimmunoassay for monitoring patients with epithelial ovarian carcinoma: Comparison of CA125 and CEA. Proc Am Soc Clin Oncol 2:6–43.

Battifera H, Trowbridge IS (1983): A monoclonal antibody useful for the differential diagnosis between malignant lymphoma and nonhematopoetic neoplasms. Cancer 51:816–821.

Bauer HW (1981): The pregnancy-associated alpha 2-glycoprotein (alpha2-PAG): A tumour marker? Klin Wochenschr 59:149–155.

Becker D, Lanse MA, Cooper GM (1982): Identification of an antigen associated with transforming genes of human and mouse mammary carcinomas. Proc Natl Acad Sci USA 79:3315–3319.

Beckstead JH (1983): Alkaline phosphatase histochemistry in human germ cell neoplasms. Am J Surg Pathol 7:341–349.

Begent RH, Green AJ, Searle F, Keep PA, Bagshawe KD, Jones BE, Jewkes RF (1983): The value of radioimmunodetection with antibody to CEA in the management of recurrent colorectal cancer. Proc Am Assoc Cancer Res 23:801.

Belitsky P, Ghose T, Aquino J, Norvell ST, Blair AH (1978): Radionuclide imaging of primary renal-cell carcinoma by I-131-labeled antitumor antibody. J Nucl Med 19:427–430.

Bell CE Jr. (1976): A normal adult and fetal lung antigen present at different quantitative levels in different histologic types of human lung cancer. Cancer 37:706–713.

Bell CE Jr, Seetharam S (1976): A plasma membrane antigen highly associated with oat-cell carcinoma of the lung and undetectable in normal adult tissue. Int J Cancer 18:605–611.

Bell DA, Flotte TJ (1982): Factor VIII related antigen in adenomatoid tumors. Implications for histogenesis. Cancer 50:932–938.

Bell H (1982): Alpha-fetoprotein and carcinoembryonic antigen in patients with primary liver carcinoma, metastatic liver disease, and alcoholic liver disease. Scand J Gastroenterol 17:897–903.

Bellet DH, Wands JR, Isselbacher KJ, Bohuon C (1984): Serum alpha-fetoprotein levels in human disease: Perspective from a highly specific monoclonal radioimmunoassay. Proc Natl Acad Sci USA 81:3869–3873.

Berche C, Mach JP, Lumbroso JD, Langlais C, Aubry F, Buchegger F, Carrel S, Rougier P, Parmentier C, Tubiana M (1982): Tomoscintigraphy for detecting gastrointestinal and medullary thyroid cancers: First clinical result using radiolabeled monoclonal antibodies against carcinoembryonic antigen. Br Med J 285:1447–1451.

Berg K, Noer G, Stavem P (1977): Human leukemia associated antigen (LAA): Occurrence and characteristics. Scand J Haematol 19:463–469.

Berger C, Takezaki S, DePietro W, Chu A, Morrison S, Edelson R. (1981):Production of monoclonal antibodies reactive with the neoplastic lymphocytes of cutaneous T cell lymphoma. J Invest Dermatol 76:311.

Berger CL, Morrison S, Chu A, Patterson J, Estabrook A, Takezaki S, Sharon J, Warburton D, Irigoyen O, Edelson RL (1982): Diagnosis of cutaneous T-cell lymphoma by use of monoclonal antibodies reactive with tumor-associated antigens. J Clin Invest 70:1205–1215.

Bergstrand CG, Czar B (1956): Demonstration of a new protein in serum from human fetus. Scand J Clin Lab Invest 8:174.

Berkman JI, Mesa-Tejada R, Klavins JV, Weiss M (1975): Demonstration of cross-reacting human tumor antigens by immunoperoxidase staining techniques. Fed Proc 34:834.

Bernal SD, Speak JA (1984): Membrane antigen in small cell carcinoma of the lung defined by monoclonal antibody SM2. Cancer Res. 44:265–270.
Bhattacharya M, Barlow J (1973): Immunologic studies of human serous cystadenocarcinoma of ovary: Demonstration of tumor-associated antigens. Cancer 31:588–595.
Bhattacharya M, Chatterjee SK (1980): Antigen(s) markers in ovarian cancer. Proc Am Assoc Cancer Res 21:216.
Bhattacharya, M, Barlow JJ, Chu TM, Piver MS (1974): Tumor-associated antigen(s) from granulosa cell carcinomas of the ovary. Cancer Res 34:812–822.
Billing R, Terasaki PI (1974): Human leukemia antigen. II. Purification. J Natl Cancer Inst 53:1639–1643.
Billing R, Minowada J, Cline M, Clark B, Lee K (1978): Acute lymphocytic leukemia-associated cell membrane antigen. J Natl Cancer Inst 61:423–429.
Billing R, Lucero K, Shi BJ, Terasaki PI (1982): A new acute leukemia-associated blast cell antigen detected by a monoclonal antibody. Blood 59:1203–1206.
Birdi A, Gupta S, Gambhir SS (1984): Plasma histaminase activity in carcinoma of the cervix—its clinical significance. J Surg Oncol 25:296–299.
Birkmayer GD, Stass H-P (1980): Humoral immune response in glioma patients: A solubilized glioma-associated membrane antigen as a tool for detecting circulating antibodies. Int J Cancer 25:445–452.
Birkmayer GD, Miller F, Marguth F (1974a): Oncornaviral information in human glioblastoma. J Neurol Transm 35:241–254.
Birkmayer GD, Balda B-R, Miller F (1974b): Oncornaviral information in human melanoma. Eur J Cancer 10:419–424.
Bizzari JP, Mackillop WJ, Buick RN (1983): Cellular specificity of NB70K, a putative human ovarian tumor antigen. Cancer Res 43:864–867.
Björklund B, Björklund V (1957): Antigenicity of pooled human malignant and normal tissues by cyto-immunological technique: Presence of an insoluble, heat-labile tumor antigen. Int Arch Allergy 10:153–184.
Björklund V, Björklund B, Wittekind C, von Kleist S (1982): Immuno-histochemical localization of tissue polypeptide antigen (TPA) and carcino-embryonic antigen (CEA) in breast cancer. Acta Pathol Microbiol Immunol Scand 90:471–476.
Bloom ET (1977): Antigen(s) on human transitional cell carcinoma detected by a xenogeneic antiserum. Urol Res 5:141–148.
Bloomer JR (1980): Serum alpha-fetoprotein in nonneoplastic liver-diseases. Digest Dis Sci 25:241–242.
Blumenfeld Z, Kerner H, Thaler I, Deutsch M, Beck D (1984): Increased alpha-fetoprotein levels in mixed mesodermal tumor of the ovary. Gynecol Obstet Invest 17:169–173.
Body JJ, Heath Hd (1984): "Nonspecific" increase in plasma immunoreactive calcitonin in healthy individuals: Discrimination from medullary thyroid carcinoma by a new extraction technique. Clin Chem 30:511–514.
Boland CR, Montgomery CK, Kim YS (1982): Alterations in human colonic mucin occurring with cellular differentiation and malignant transformation. Proc Natl Acad Sci USA 79:2051–2055.
Boon ME, Lindeman J, Meeuwissen AL, Otto AJ (1982): Carcinoembryonic antigen in sputum cytology. Acta Cytol 26:389–394.
Borek E, Waalkes TP, Gehrke CH (1983): Tumor markers derived from nucleic acid components. In Nieburgs HE, Birkmayer GD, Klavins JV (eds): "Human Tumor Markers: Biological Basis and Clinical Relevance." New York: Alan R. Liss, pp 67–71.
Braatz JA, Hua DT, Princler GL (1983): Serum levels of a human lung tumor-associated antigen using an improved radioimmunoassay. Cancer Res 43:110–113.

Bradstock KF, Janossy G, Hoffbrand AV, Ganeshaguru K, Llewellin P, Prentice HG, Bollum FJ (1981): Immunofluorescent and biochemical studies of terminal deoxynucleotidyl transferase in treated acute leukaemia. Br J Haematol 47:121–131.

Bradwell AR, Fairweather DS, Dykes PW (1983): Detection of tumours using radiolabeled antibodies. Radiography 49:5–12.

Braunstein GD, Vaitukaitis JL, Carbone PP, Ross GT (1973): Ectopic production of human chorionic gonadotropin by neoplasms. Ann Intern Med 78:39–45.

Bray J, McPherson TA (1981): Fc receptor-bearing peripheral blood mononuclear cells in breast cancer patients: A possible marker of tumor burden and prognosis. Clin Exp Immunol 44:629–637.

Brenckman WD, Lastinger LB, Sedor F (1981): Unpredictable fluctuations in serum acid phosphatase activity in prostatic cancer. JAMA 245:2501–2504.

Brenner BG, Jothy S, Shuster J, Fuks A (1982): Monoclonal antibodies of human lung tumor antigens demonstrated by immunofluorescence and immunoprecipitation. Cancer Res 42:3187–3192.

Brichacek B, Hirsch I, Sibi O, Vilikusova E, Vonka V (1983): Association of some supraglottic laryngeal carcinomas with EB virus. Int J Cancer 32:193–197.

Brockamp G, Braun J, Langer S (1982): The value of carcinoembryonic antigen and Tennessee antigen in diagnosis of rectal carcinoma. Aktuel Chir 17:99–101.

Brodeur GM, Seeger RC, Schwab M, Varmus HE, Bishop JM (1984): Amplification of N-myc in untreated human neuroblastomas with advanced disease stage. Science 224:1121–1124.

Brown G, Netzel B, Thiel E, Hoffman-Fezer G, Thierfelder S (1979): Characterization of antigens on acute lymphoblastic leukemias. Haematol Blood Transfus 23:365–368.

Brown JP, Nishiyama K, Hellström I, Hellström KE (1981a): Structural characterization of human melanoma-associated antigen p97 with monoclonal antibodies. J Immunol 127:539–546.

Brown JP, Woodbury RG, Hart CE, Hellström I, Hellström KE (1981b): Quantitative analysis of melanoma-associated antigen p97 in normal and neoplastic tissues. Proc Natl Acad Sci USA 78:539–543.

Brown SE, Howard CR, Steward MW, Ajdukiewicz AB, Whittle HC (1984): Hepatitis B surface antigen containing immune complexes occur in seronegative hepatocellular carcinoma patients. Clin Exp Immunol 55:355–359.

Bubenik J (1975): Cell-mediated tumour immunity in patients with transitional cell carcinoma of the urinary bladder. Int Urol Nephrol 7:297–302.

Bucovaz ET, Morrison JC, Whybrew WD, Macleod RM, Wakim JM, Fryer JE (1978): B-protein assay: Protein-protein interaction used to detect a serum protein present in individuals with cancer. Fed Proc 37:1282.

Buffe D, Rimbaut C (1975): H-globulin, a hepatic glycoferroprotein: Characterization and clinical significance. Ann NY Acad Sci 259:417–426.

Burtin P, Gendron MC (1973): A tumor-associated antigen in human nephroblastoma. Proc Natl Acad Sci USA 70:2051–2054.

Busch H, Busch RK, Chan PK, Isenberg W, Weigand R, Russo J, Furmanski P (1981): Results of a preliminary "blind" study on the presence of the human tumor nucleolar antigen in breast carcinomas, benign breast tumors, and normal breast tissues. Clin Immunol Immunopathol 18:155–167.

Busnardo B, Girelli ME, Pellizzo MR, Zorat PL, DeBasi P, Eccher C (1983): Different diagnostic significance of carcinoembryonic antigen vs calcitonin as tumor markers of medullary thyroid carcinoma. Acta Endocrinol (Copenh) Suppl 252:57–58.

Busnardo B, Girelli ME, Simioni N, Nacamulli D, Busetto E (1984): Nonparallel patterns of calcitonin and carcinoembryonic antigen levels in the follow-up of medullary thyroid carcinoma. Cancer 53:278–285.

Bychkov V, Rothman M, Bardawil WA (1983): Immunocytochemical localization of carcinoembryonic antigen (CEA), alpha-fetoprotein (AFP), and human chorionic gonadotropin (HCG) in cervical neoplasia. Am J Clin Pathol 79:414–420.

Byers VS, Hackett AJ, Riggs JL (1976): Assay for tumor specific transfer factor produced in vitro against human breast carcinoma. Proc Am Assoc Cancer Res 17:216.

Bystryn JC, Tedholm CA (1981): Shedding of human melanoma associated antigens (MAA) with plasma membrane fragments. Fed Proc 40:981.

Cabnal P, Bugat R, Soula G, Combes PF (1981): Determination of circulating ectopic beta HCG in solid tumors. Pathol Biol 29:150–154.

Cabral GA, Marciano-Cabral F, Fry D, Lumpkin CK, Mercer L, Goplerud D (1982): Expression of herpes simplex virus type 2 antigens in premalignant and malignant human vulvar cells. Am J Obstet Gynecol 143:611–619.

Cabral GA, Fry D, Marciano-Cabral F, Lumpkin C, Mercer L, Goplerud D (1983): A herpes virus antigen in human premalignant and malignant cervical biopsies and explants. Am J Obstet Gynecol 145:79–86.

Caffier H, Brandau H (1983): Serum tumor markers in metastatic breast cancer and course of disease. Cancer Det Prev 6:451–457.

Cahan LD, Irie RF, Singh R, Cassidenti A, Paulson JC (1982): Identification of a human neuroectodermal tumor antigen (OFA-I-2) as ganglioside GD2. Proc Natl Acad Sci USA 79:7629–7633.

Callahan R, Drohan W, Tronick S, Schlom J (1982): Detection and cloning of human DNA sequences related to mouse mammary tumor virus genome. Proc Natl Acad Sci USA 79:5503–5507.

Calmettes C, Moukhtar MS, Milhaud G (1978): Plasma carcinoembryonic antigen versus plasma calcitonin in the diagosis of medullary carcinoma of the thyroid. Cancer Immunol Immunother 4:251–256.

Calmettes C, Caillou B, Moukhtar MS, Milhaud G, Gerard-Marchant R (1982): Calcitonin and carcinoembryonic antigen in poorly differentiated follicular carcinoma. Cancer 49:2342–2348.

Capel ID, Dorrell HM, Williams DC, Hanham IWF, Levitt HN (1982): Serum galactosyl transferase levels in patients with advanced cancer. Oncology 39:193–196.

Capon DJ, Seeburg PH, McGrath JP, Hayflick JS, Edman U, Levinson AD, Goeddel DV (1983): Activation of Ki-ras2 gene in human colon and lung carcinomas by two different point mutations. Nature 304:507–513.

Carachi R, Beeley JG (1983): Polyamines in colorectal cancer—a clinical and experimental approach. J Clin Pathol 36:508–510.

Carlsson U, Stewenius J, Ekelund G, Leandoor L, Nosslin B (1983): Is CEA analysis of value in screening for recurrence after surgery for colorectal carcinoma? Dis Colon Rectum 26:369–373.

Cassareale D, Sakamoto K, Aiba M, Katayama I, Purtilo DT, Humphreys RE (1981): Sera of patients with hairy cell leukemia immunoprecipitate EBV-related antigens. Leuk Res 5:107–112.

Catalano LW Jr, Harter DH, Hsu KC (1972): Common antigen in meningioma-derived cell cultures. Science 175:180–182.

Catalano WJ, Menon M (1981): New screening and diagnostic tests for prostate cancer and immunologic assessment. Urology 17:61–65.

Cazzola N, Arioso P, Gobbi PG, Barosi G, Bergamaschi G, Dezza L, Iacobello C, Ascari E (1983): Basic and acidic isoferritins in the serum of patients with Hodgkin's disease. Eur J Cancer Clin Oncol 19:339–345.

Chan JS, Seidah NG, Chretien M (1983): Human NH_2 terminal of pro-opiomelanocortin as a potential marker for pulmonary carcinoma. Cancer Res 43:3066–3069.

Chan PK, Frakes R, Tan EM, Brattain MG, Smetana K, Busch H (1983): Indirect immunofluorescence studies of proliferating cell nuclear antigen in nucleoli of human tumor and normal tissues. Cancer Res 43:3770–3777.

Chattopadhyay SK, Chang EH, Lander MR, Ellis RW, Scolnick EM, Lowy DR (1982): Amplification and rearrangement of onc gene in mammalian species. Nature 296:361–363.

Chawla RK, Heymsfield SB, Wadsworth AA, Shoji M, Rudman D (1977): Isolation and characterization of a glycoprotein (JBBS) in the urine of a patient with carcinoma of the colon. Cancer Res 37:873–878.

Chayen D, Chayen R, Dvir R, Goldberg S, Harell A, Lichtenstein D, Stavorovsky M (1983): Urinary excretion of spermine in breast cancer. Adv Polyamine Res 4:65–72.

Chechik BE, Percy ME, Gelfand EW (1978): Human thymus-leukemia-associated antigen: Isolation and partial characterization. J Natl Cancer Inst 60:69–75.

Chechik BE, Jason J, Shore A, Baker M, Dosch H-M, Gelfand EW (1979): Quantitation of human thymus/leukemia-associated antigen by radioimmunoassay in different forms of leukemia. Blood 54:1400–1406.

Chen D-S, Sung J-L, Sheu J-C, Lai M-Y, How S-W, Hsu H-C, Lee C-S, Wei T-C (1984): Serum α-fetoprotein in the early stage of human hepatocellular carcinoma. Gastroenterology 86:1404–1409.

Cheresh DA, Reisfeld RA, Varki AP (1984): O-Acetylation of disialoganglioside GD_3 by human melanoma cells creates a unique antigenic determinant. Science 225:844–846.

Cherubini M, Agonegro M, Delbello A, Visintin A, Trani S, Mattiussi A (1982): Carcinoma of the rectum and importance of haptoglobin as a diagnostic marker (Multivariate analysis of acute-phase reactive proteins in surgery). Acta Chir Ital 38:238–249.

Child JA, Crawford SM, Norfolk DR, O'Quigly J, Scarfe JH, Struthers LP (1983): Evaluation of serum beta 2-microglobulin as a prognostic indicator in myelomatosis. Br J Cancer 47:111–114.

Chin J, Miller F (1984): Murine monoclonal antibodies to a human pancreatic adenocarcinoma-associated antigen. Fed Proc 43:1513.

Chiu J-F, Hnilica LS, Chytil F, Orrahood JT, Rogers LW (1977): Tissue-specific antibodies against human lung and breast carcinoma dehistonized chromatins. J Natl Cancer Inst 59:151–154.

Chu TM, Bhargaca A, Barnard EA, Ostrowski W, Varkarakis MJ, Merrin C, Murphy GP (1975): Tumor antigen and acid phosphatase isoenzyme in prostatic cancer. Cancer Chemother Rep 59:97–103.

Chu TM, Holyoke ED, Douglass HD (1977): Isolation of a glycoprotein antigen from ascites fluid of pancreatic carcinoma. Cancer Res 37:1525–1529.

Chung WK, Sun HS, Park DH, Minuk GY, Hoofnagle JH (1983): Primary hepatocellular carcinoma and hepatitis B virus infection in Korea. J Med Virol 11:99–104.

Cleary MC, Chao J, Warnke R, Sklar J (1984): Immunoglobulin gene rearrangement as a diagnostic criterion of B-cell lymphoma. Proc Natl Acad Sci USA 81:593–597.

Coakham HB, Lakshmi MS (1975): Tumour-associated surface antigen(s) in human astrocytomas. Oncology 31:233–243.

Cocchia D, Lauriola L, Stolfi VM, Tallini G, Michetti F (1983): S-100 antigen labels neoplastic cells in liposarcoma and cartilaginous tumours. Virchows Arch 402:139–145.

Cochran AJ, Grant RM, Spilg WG, Mackie RM, Ross CE, Hoyle DE, Russell JM (1974): Sensitization to tumour-associated antigens in human breast carcinoma. Int J Cancer 14:19–25.

Cochran AJ, Todd G, Hart DM, Morrison LJ, Mackie RM (1982): Reaction of the leukocytes of melanoma patients and control donors, including pregnant women, with melanoma-and fetus-derived materials. Cancer Immunol Immunother 14:78–81.

Coggin JH Jr, Payne WJ (1984): The development and detection of mouse monoclonal antibody to embryonic antigen on rodent and human fetus and on tumor cells. Proc Am Assoc Cancer Res 25:271.

Cohen AM, Ketcham AS, Morton DL (1973): Tumor-specific cellular cytotoxicity to human sarcomas: Evidence for cell-mediated host immune response to a sarcoma cell-surface antigen. J Natl Cancer Inst 50:585–589.

Collins S, Groudine M (1982): Amplification of endogenous myc-related DNA sequences in a human myeloid leukemia cell line. Nature 298:679–681.

Collins SJ, Kubonishi I, Miyoshi I, Groudine MT (1984): Altered transcription of the c-abl oncogene in K-562 and other chronic myelogenous leukemia cells. Science 225:72–74.

Colombi M, Barlati S, Magdelenat H, Fiszer-Szarfaz B (1984): Relationship between multiple forms of plasminogen activator in human breast tumors and plasma and the presence of metastases in lymph nodes. Cancer Res 44:2971–2975.

Coon JS, Weinstein RS, Summers JL (1982): Blood group precursor T-antigen expression in human urinary bladder carcinoma. Am J Clin Pathol 77:692–699.

Copeman PWM, Cooke KB (1979): Significance of malignant melanoma antigen (melanoma specific protein) in the urine. J Roy Soc Med 72:95–99.

Coppack S, Newlands ES, Dent J, Michell H, Goka G, Bagshawe KD (1983): Problems of interpretation of serum concentrations of alpha-fetoprotein (AFP) in patients receiving cytotoxic chemotherapy for malignant germ cell tumour. Br J Cancer 48:335–340.

Cordes U, Rothmund M, Eberle S, Krause U, Kolbe K, Braun B, Reinsdorf S, Beyer J (1983): Carcinoembryonic antigen determination in the differentiation of pheochromocytoma with ectopic calcitonin formation and multiple endocrine neoplasia Type II. Dtsch Med Wochenschr 108:462–464.

Corson JM, Pinkus GS (1982): Mesothelioma: Profile of keratin proteins and carcinoembryonic antigen, an immunoperoxidase study of 20 cases and comparison with pulmonary adenocarcinomas. Am J Pathol 108:80–88.

Cortes EP, Chu TM, Wang JJ, Holyoke D, Wallace HJ, Murphy GP (1977): Carcinoembryonic antigen in osteosarcoma. J Surg Oncol 9:257–265.

Costa J, Howley PM, Bowling MC, Howard R, Bauer WC (1981): Presence of human papilloma viral antigens in juvenile multiple laryngeal papilloma. Am J Clin Pathol 75:194–197.

Crawford IV, Pim DC, Bulbrook (1982): Detection of antibodies against the cellular protein p53 in sera from patients with breast cancer. Int J Cancer 30:403–408.

Crepin M, Lidereau R, Chermann JC, Pouillart P, Magdelenat H, Montagnier L (1984): Sequences related to mouse mammary tumor virus genome in tumor cells and lymphocytes from patients with breast cancer. Biochem Biophys Res Commun 118:324–331.

Criss WE (1971): A review of isoenzymes in cancer. Cancer Res 31:1523–1542.

Croce CM (1984): Chromosome translocations and c-myc oncogene activation in Burkitt lymphoma. Fed Proc 43:6.

Croghan GA, Wingate MB, Gamarrra M, Johnson E, Chu TM, Allen H, Valenzuela L, Tsukada Y, Papsidero LD (1984): Reactivity of monoclonal antibody F36/22 with human ovarian adenocarcinomas. Cancer Res 44:1954–1962.

Cuatico W, Cho J-R, Spiegelman S (1973): Particles with RNA-directed DNA polymerase in human brain tumors. Proc Natl Acad Sci USA 70:2789–2793.

Cuttitta F, Rosen S, Gazdar AF, Minna JD (1981): Monoclonal antibodies that demonstrate specificity for general types of human lung cancer. Proc Natl Acad Sci USA 78:4591–4595.

Dahlmann N, Pompecki R (1984): Human serum deoxythymidine-5′-triphosphatase activity as a parameter in the diagnosis and follow-up of large bowel carcinoma. Cancer Res 44:848–851.

Dalifard I, Davor A, Cellier P, Larra F (1984): What value should be given to assays of serum ferritin in breast cancers? Correlation with various biological parameters. Sem Hop Paris 60:157–162.

Damjanov I, Amenta PS, Zarghami F (1984): Transformation of an AFP-positive yolk sac carcinoma into an AFP-negative neoplasm. Evidence for in vivo cloning of the human parietal yolk sac carcinoma. Cancer 53:1902–1907.

Damjanov I, Fox N, Knowles BB, Solter D, Lange PH, Fraley EE (1982): Immunohistochemical localization of murine stage-specific embryonic antigens in human testicular germ cell tumors. Am J Pathol 108:225–230.

Danon YL, Seeger RC, Maidman JE (1980): Fetal neural antigens on human neuroblastoma cells. J Immunol 124:2925–2929.

Das A, Roy IS, Maitra TK, Kanjilal A (1984): Significance of carcinoembryonic antigen in retinoblastoma. Br J Ophthalmol 68:252–254.

Dash RJ, Dutta RK, Sharma BA, Sehgal L (1979): Serum alpha-fetoprotein in non-hepatic malignancies. Indian J Med Res 70:980–985.

Davey RA, Harvie RM, Cahill EJ, Levi JA (1984): Serum galactosyltransferase isoenzymes as markers for solid tumours in humans. Eur J Cancer Clin Oncol 20:75–79.

Davies SN, Gochman N (1983): Evaluation of a monoclonal antibody-based immunoradiometric assay for prostatic acid phosphatase. Am J Clin Pathol 79:114–119.

Davis FM, Hittelmann WN, McCredie KB, Keating MJ, Vellekoop L, Rao PN (1984): Human malignancy-associated nucleolar antigen or a marker for tumor cells in patients with acute leukemia. Blood 63:676–683.

Dayal Y, O'Briain DS, Nunnemacher G, DeLellis RA, Wolfe HJ, Reichlin S (1982): Somatostatin as a marker for carcinoid tumors: An immunohistochemical and ultrastructural study. Lab Invest 46:17A.

Debus E, Moll R, Frankl WW, Weber K, Osborn M (1984): Immunohistochemical distinction of human carcinomas by cytokeratin typing with monoclonal antibodies. Am J Pathol 114:121–130.

DeFazio RS, Gozzo JJ, Monaco AP (1982): Tumor-associated antigens in the urine of patients with bladder cancer. Cancer Res 42:2913–2917.

DeLong Bolmer S, Davidson EA (1981): Preparation and properties of a glycoprotein associated with malignancy. Biochemistry 20:1047–1054.

Delpech B, Delpech A, Girard N, Chauzy C, Laumonier R (1978): A mesenchymal antigen: A new immunochemical marker of human tumors. CR Acad Sci (Paris) 287:1351–1352.

Del Villano BC, Brennan S, Brock P, Bucher C, Liu V, McClure M, Rake B, Space S, Westrick B, Schoemaker H, Zurawski VR (1983): Radioimmunometric assay for a monoclonal antibody-defined tumor marker, Ca19-9. Clin Chem 29:549–552.

De Mello J, Leveson SH, Wiggins PA, Highley B, Cooper EH, Giles GR (1982): The detection of gastrointestinal cancer using a panel of cancer markers. Br J Surg 69:283.

Dent PB, Liao SK, McCulloch PB, Macnamara J (1976): Melanoma antigens on cultured melanoma cell lines detected by xeno- and alloantibody. Proc Am Soc Clin Oncol 17:311.

Der, CJ, Cooper GM (1983): Altered gene products are associated with activation of cellular *ras*-K genes in human lung and colon carcinomas. Cell 32:201–208.

Deutsch E, Apffel CA, Mori H, Walker JE (1973): A tumor-associated antigen in gastric cancer secretions. Cancer Res 33:112–116.

Dickinson JP, Smith JH, Dyson JED (1976): A cell surface antigen common to human tumours: Detection, localization and characterization. Biochem Soc Trans 4:125–127.

Dillmann E, Lopez-Karpovitch X, Alvarez-Hernandez X, Hurtado R, Cordova MS, Gonzalez-Llaven J, Diaz Maqueo JC (1982): Ferritin and malignant hemopathies. I. Ferritin in cerebrospinal fluid as an indicator of central nervous system leukemic involvement. Rev Invest Clin (Mex) 34:95–98.

Dion AS, Farwell DC, Pomenti AA, Girard AJ (1980): A human protein related to the major envelope protein of murine mammary tumor virus: Identification and characterization. Proc Natl Acad Sci USA 77:1301–1305.

Dippold WG, Lloyd KO, Li LT, Ikeda H, Oettgen HF, Old LJ (1980): Cell antigens of human malignant melanoma: Definition of six antigenic systems with mouse monoclonal antibodies. Proc Natl Acad Sci USA 77:6114–6118.

Dmochowski L, Ohtsuki Y (1979): Virus associated cell transformation and host alteration. Cancer Det Prev 2:531–563.

Dnistrian AM, Schwarts MK, Katopodis N, Fracchia AA, Stock CC (1982): Serum lipid-bound sialic acid as a marker in breast cancer. Cancer 50:1815–1819.

Dobrovolskii NM, Medvedev VN, Firsova PP, Filatov PP, Kosinova MV (1983): Prognostic significance of the determination of carcinoembryonic antigen in the blood of patients with lung cancer. Vopr Onkol 29:57–60.

Doellgast GJ, Homesley HD (1984): Placental-type alkaline phosphatase in ovarian cancer fluids and tissues. Obstet Gynecol 63:324–329.

Donaldson ES, van Nageli JR Jr, Gay EC, Purcell S, Meeker, WR, Kashmiri R, Hunter L, van de Voorde J. (1979): α Fetoprotein as a biochemical marker in patients with gynecologic malignancy. Gynecol Oncology 7:18–24.

Dörn MH, Abel U, Fritze D, Manke H-G, Drings P (1983): Serum ferritin in relation to the course of Hodgkin's disease. Cancer 52:2308–2312.

Dorsett, BH, Ioachim HL, Stolbach L, Walker J, Barber HRK (1975): Isolation of tumor-specific antibodies from effusions of ovarian carcinomas. Int J Cancer 16:779–786.

Drewinko B, Montgomery CT, Trujillo JM (1973): Demonstration of common sarcoma-associated antigen(s) in an established human neurogenic sarcoma cell line. Cancer Res 33:601–605.

Drexler HG, Gaedicke G, Minowada J (1984): Enzyme markers in acute leukemias: Advances during the last decade. J Natl Cancer Inst 72:1283–1298.

Drysdale JW, Alpert E (1975): Carcinofetal human isoferritins. Ann NY Acad Sci 259:427–434.

Dufek V, Matous B, Kral V (1984): Serum alkaline-stable acid thiol proteinase—a possible marker for primary liver carcinoma. Neoplasma 31:99–107.

Durante F (1874): Nesso fisio-patologico tra la struttura dei nei materni e la genesi di alcuni tumori maligni. Arch di Mem de Osservaz di Chirug Pract 11:217–226.

Duttagupta C, Romney SL, Palan PR, Slagle NS (1982): Urinary cyclic nucleotides and the cytopathology of human uterine cervical dysplasias. Cancer Res 42:2938–2943.

Dvorak HF, Van De Water L, Dvorak AM, Harvey VS, Anderson D, DeWolf W, Bach R (1982): Human tumor cells and guinea pig macrophages shed plasma membrane derived vesicles with precoagulant activity (PCA). Fed Proc 41:270.

Dyson JL, Walker PG, Singer A (1984): Human papillomavirus infection of the uterine cervix: Histological appearances in 28 cases identified by immunohistochemical techniques. J Clin Pathol 37:126–130.

Edwards JJ, Anderson NG, Tollaksen SL, von Eschenbach AC, Guevara J (1982): Proteins of human urine. II. Identification by two-dimensional electrophoresis of a new candidate marker for prostatic cancer. Clin Chem 28:160–163.

Edynak EM, Old, LJ, Vrana M, Lardis MP (1972): A fetal antigen associated with human neoplasia. N Engl J Med 286:1178–1183.

Eglin RP, Sharp F, MacLean AB, Macnab JC, Clements JB, Wilkie NM (1981): Detection of RNA complementary to herpes simplex virus DNA in human cervical squamous cell neoplasms. Cancer Res 41:3597–3603.

Elliott AY, Fraley EE, Cleveland P, Castro AE, Stein N (1973): Isolation of RNA virus from papillary tumors of the human renal pelvis. Science 179:393–395.

Elliott PG, Thurlow B, Needham PRG, Lewis MG (1973): The specificity of the cytoplasmic antigen in human malignant melanoma. Eur J Cancer 9:607–610.

Embleton MJ, Heidelberger C (1975): Neoantigens on chemically transformed cloned C3H mouse embryo cells. Cancer Res 35:2049–2055.

Embleton MJ, Price MR (1978): Detection and partial purification of melanoma-associated antigen. Br J Dermatol 99:19.

Embleton MJ, Gunn B, Byers VS, Baldwin RW (1981): Antitumour reactions of monoclonal antibody against a human osteogenic-sarcoma cell line. Br J Cancer 43:582–587.

Endrizzi L, Fiorentino MV, Salvagno L, Segati R, Pappagallo GL, Fosser V (1982): Serum lactate dehydrogenase (LDH) as a prognostic index for non-Hodgkin's lymphoma. Eur J Cancer Clin Oncol 18:945–949.

Espinoza CG, Saba SR, Shelley SA, Paciga JE, Balis JV (1982): Antibodies to surfactant "apoprotein" as a diagnostic tool for identifying carcinomas of the lung with associated alveolar cell differentiation. Lab Invest 46:21A.

Eusebi V, Bondi A, Rosai J (1984): Immunohistochemical localization of myoglobin in nonmuscular cells. Am J Surg Pathol 8:51–55.

Faravelli B, D'Amore E, Nosenzo M, Betta PG, Donna A (1984): Carcinoembryonic antigen in pleural effusions. Diagnostic value in malignant mesothelioma. Cancer 53:1194–1197.

Favre R, Carcassonne Y, Meyer G (1978): A surface antigen associated with Hodgkin's disease: Brief communication. J Natl Cancer Inst 59:1727–1730.

Federman JL, Lewis MG, Clark WH (1974): Tumor-associated antibodies to ocular and cutaneous malignant melanomas: Negative interaction with normal choroidal melanocytes. J Natl Cancer Inst 52:587–589.

Feickert HJ, Rettig W, Real FX, Chorney K, Anger B, Cordon-Cardo C, Melamed MR, Takahaski T, Lloyd KO, Oettgen HF, Old LJ (1983): Cell surface antigens of non-small cell lung cancer (NSCL) defined by monoclonal antibodies. Proc Am Assoc Cancer Res 23:890.

Feig LA, Bast RC Jr, Knapp RC, Cooper GM (1984): Somatic activation of ras^K gene in a human ovarian carcinoma. Science 223:698–701.

Feinberg AP, Vogelstein B, Droller MJ, Baylin SB, Nelkin BD (1983): Mutation affecting the 12th amino acid of the c-Ha-ras oncogene product occurs infrequently in human cancer. Science 220:1175–1177.

Feit C, Bartal AH, Hirshaut Y (1982): The use of monoclonal antibodies for the detection of human connective tissue differentiation antigens appearing on sarcomas. Hybridoma 1:203.

Fellous M, Bono R, Hyafil F, Gresser I, (1981): Interferon enhances the amount of membrane-bound beta2-microglobulin and its release from human Burkitt cells. Eur J Immunol 11:524–526.

Fett JW, Holton OD, Alderman EM, Goust JM, Lovins RE (1978): Characterization of antigen and antibody in human breast cancer. Clin Res 26:376.

Finn O, Gaillard M, Lam M, Zeleznik N, Hollingsworth M, Mahvi D, Metzgar R (1984): Antigens of human pancreatic tumors. Fed Proc 43:1419.

Fish RG (1973): A possible in-vitro blood test for cancer. Lancet 2:670

Fishman WH (1980): Tumor markers in neoplasia. Cancer Bull 32:45–47

Fishman WH, Inglis NR, Green S (1971): Regan isoenzyme: A carcinoplacental antigen. Cancer Res 31:1054–1057.

Foon K, Bunn P, Schroff A, Mayer D, Sherwin S, Longe D, Ochs J, Bottino G, Fer M, Herberman R, Oldham R (1983): Monoclonal antibody therapy of chronic lymphocytic leukemia (CLL) and cutaneous T-cell lymphoma (CTCL). Proc Am Soc Clin Oncol 2:C–188.

Ford CH, Newman CE, Johnson JR, Woodhouse CS, Reeder TA, Rowland GF, Simmonds RG (1983): Localization and toxicity study of a vindesine-anti-CEA conjugate in patients with advanced cancer. Br J Cancer 47:35–42.

Ford CHZ, Newman CE (1979): Expression of a cross-reactive foetal antigen in lung cancer. Clin Oncol 5:387–388.

Ford RJ, Cramer M, Davis FM (1984): Identification of human lymphoma cells by antigen to malignancy-associated nucleolar antigens. Blood 63:559–565.

Fossati G, Canevari S, Porta GD, Balzarini GP, Veronesi U (1972): Cellular immunity to human breast carcinoma. Int J Cancer 10:391–396.

Fowler JE Jr, Sesterheen I, Stutzman RE, Mostofi FK (1983): Localization of alpha-fetoprotein and human chorionic gonadotropin to specific histologic types of nonseminomatous testicular cancer. Urology 22:649–654.

Fox JN, Sheikh KM, Gupta RK, Rea TH, Morton DL, Levan NE (1981): Melanoma: Associated antigens in benign melanocytic disorders. Int J Dermatol 20:368–373.

Fox N, Damjanov I, Knowles BB, Solter D (1983): Immunohistochemical localization of the mouse stage-specific embryonic antigen 1 in human tissues and tumors. Cancer Res 43:669–678.

Franchimont P, Bouffioux C, Reuter A, Rigo-Betz C, Vrindts-Gevaert Y, Jaspar JM, Lecomte-Yerna MJ (1983): Radioimmunoassay of prostatic acid phosphatase: Validation and clinical application. Int J Cancer 31:149–155.

Fritsche R, Mach JP (1975): Identification of a new oncofetal antigen associated with several types of human carcinomas. Nature 258:734–737.

Fritze D, Kern DH, Drogemuller CR, Pilch YH (1976): Production of antisera with specificity for malignant melanoma and human fetal skin. Cancer Res 36:458–466.

Froelich TW, Buchanan G, Cornet JM, Sartain PA, Smith RG (1981): Terminal deoxynucleotidyl transferase-containing cells in peripheral blood: Implications for the surveillance of patients with lymphoblastic leukemia or lymphoma in remission. Blood 58:214–220.

Frost MJ, Rogers GT, Bagshawe KD (1975): Extraction and preliminary characterization of a human bronchogenic carcinoma antigen. Br J Cancer 31:379–386.

Fukuda M (1980a): K562 human leukaemic cells express fetal type (i) antigen on different glycoproteins from circulating erythrocytes. Nature 285:405–407.

Fukuda M (1980b): The leukocyte migration inhibition test on tumor associated antigens in breast cancer patients. Nippon Geka Gakkai Zasshi 81:1423–1436.

Furukawa K, Takizawa H, Iseki S (1977): Immunochemical studies on human cancer. I. Cancer-associated antigen reacting with anti-stomach cancer immune serum. Proc Jpn Acad 53:161–166.

Gaffar SA, Braatz JA, Kortright KH, Princler GL, McIntire KR (1979): Further studies on a human lung tumor-associated antigen. Comparison of antigens from different tumors. J Biol Chem 254:2097–2102.

Gallo RC (1976): New molecular biological findings on subviral components related to primate carcinogenic RNA tumor viruses in human leukemia. In: Deutsch E, Moser K, Rainer H, Stacher A (eds): "Molecular Base of Malignancy. New Clinical and Therapeutic Evidence." Stuttgart: Georg Thieme, pp 177–178.

Gallo RC, Reitz MS (1982): Human retroviruses and adult T-cell leukemia-lymphoma. J Natl Cancer Inst 69:1209–1214.

Gallo RC, Wong-Staal F (1982): Retroviruses as etiologic agents of some animal and human leukemias and lymphomas and as tools for elucidating the molecular mechanism of leukemogenesis. Blood 60.545–557.

Gallo RC, Sarin PS, Gelmann EP, Robert-Guroff M, Richardson E, Kalyanaraman VS, Mann D, Sidhu GD, Stahl RE, Zolla-Pazner S, Leibovitch J, Popovic M (1983): Isolation of human T-cell leukemia virus in acquired immune deficiency syndrome (AIDS). Science 220:865–867.

Galloway DR, Imai K, Ferrone S, Reisfeld RA (1981): Molecular profiles of human melanoma-associated antigens. Fed Proc 40:231–236.

Galvan L, Evans JE, Comis RL, Gottlieb A, Gyorkey F, Lane M, Prestayko AW, Crooke ST (1982): Detection of a serum DNA-binding protein associated with cancer. Cancer Res 42:1562–1566.

Gangal SG, Agashe SS, Nair PNM, Rao RS, Randadive KJ (1975): Onco-fetal cross reactivity between human osteogenic sarcoma and foetal periosteal fibroblasts grown in vitro. Indian J Med 63:851–857.

Ganz PA, Shell WE, Tokes ZA (1983): Evaluation of a radioimmunoassay for alpha 1-acid glycoprotein to monitor therapy of cancer patients. J Natl Cancer Inst 71:25–30.

Garancis JC, Tieu TM, Limoni A (1983): Classification of pituitary tumors based on immunocytology and electron microscopy. Cancer Det Prev 6:595.

Gasser RW, Judmaier G, zur Nedden D, Aufschnaiter M, Hogstaedter F (1983): Primary hepatocellular carcinoma with hepatitis B virus infection in a 16-year old noncirrhotic patient. Am J Gastronenterol 78:305–308.

Gauduchon P, Tillier C, Guyonnet C, Heron JF, Bar-Guilloux E, Le Talaer JY (1983): Clinical value of serum glycoprotein galactosytransferase levels in different histological types of ovarian carcinoma. Cancer Res 43:4491–4496.

Gazitt Y, Gilead Z, Klein G, Sulitzeanu D (1981): A technique for the identification of glycoprotein antigens in immune complexes and its application to the detection of a common glycoprotein in sera of patients with Burkitt's lymphoma and nasopharyngeal carcinoma J. Immunol Methods 43:49–57.

Gazitt Y, Bentwich Z, Shani A (1983): Reactivity of purified GP40 antigen with antibodies from sera of patients colorectal cancer: A follow-up study. Int J Cancer 32:537–541.

Gelder FB, Reese C, Moossa C, Hunter RL (1979): Pancreatic oncofetal antigen. In Herberman RB, McIntire KR (eds): "Immunodiagnosis of Cancer, Vol 9" New York: Marcel Dekker, pp 357–368.

Ghazizadeh M, Kagawa S, Izumi K, Maebayashi K, Takigawa H, Saiki T, Kawano A, Kurokawa K (1984): Immunohistochemical detection of carcinoembryonic antigen in benign hyperplasia and adenocarcinoma of the prostate with monoclonal antibody. J Urol 131:501–503.

Giacomini P, Ng AK, Kantor RRS, Natali PG, Ferrone S (1983): Double determinant immunoassay to measure a human high-molecular-weight melanoma-associated antigen. Cancer Res. 43:3586–3590.

Gjerris F, Peitersen B, Nielsen K, Arends J, Haase J, Lindholm J, Wewer U, Albrechtsen R (1982): Alpha-fetoprotein (AFP) and human chorionic gonadotrophin (HCG) as tumor markers in cases of intracranial and intraspinal germ-cell tumors. Ugeskr Laeger 144: 1296–1299.

Go VL, Zamcheck N (1982): The role of tumor markers in the management of colorectal cancer. Cancer 50:2618–2623.

Gold DV (1977): Structural studies on human colonic mucoprotein antigen obtained from normal and tumoral tissues. Dis Abst Int (B) 38:2607–2608.

Gold P, Freedman S (1965): Demonstration of tumor-specific antigens in human colonic carcinomata by immunological tolerance and absorption techniques. J Exp Med 121: 439–471.

Goldenberg DM, Kim EE, Bennett SJ, Nelson MO, DeLand FH (1983a): Carcinoembryonic antigen radioimmunodetection in the evaluation of colorectal cancer and the detection of occult neoplasms. Gastroenterology 84:524–532.

Goldenberg DM, DeLand FH, Bennett SJ, Primus FJ, Nelson MO, Flanigan RC, McRoberts JW, Bruce AW, Mahan DE (1983b): Radioimmunodetection of prostatic cancer. In vivo use of radioactive antibodies against prostatic cancer by nuclear imaging. JAMA 250: 630–635.

Goldenberg DM, Sharkey RM, Primus FJ, Mizusawa E, Hawthorne MF (1984): Neutron-capture therapy of human cancer: In vivo results on tumor localization of Boron-10-labeled antibodies to carcinoembryonic antigen in the GW-39 tumor model system. Proc Natl Acad Sci USA 81:560–563.

Goldrosar MH, Dasmahapatra K, Jenkins D, Howell JH, Arbuck SG, Moore MC, Douglass HD (1981): Microplate leukocyte adherence inhibition (LAI) assay in pancreatic cancer: Detection of specific antitumor immunity with patient's peripheral blood cells and serum. Cancer 47:1614–1619.

Goodyear MD, Malkin A, Malkin DG, Sutherland DJ (1983): Relationship between estrogen (ER) and progesterone (PR) receptors and carcinoembryonic antigen (CEA) in human breast carcinoma cytosols. Proc Am Soc Clin Oncol 2:C–60.

Gordon SG (1981): A proteolytic procoagulant associated with malignant transformation. J Histochem Cytochem 219:457–463.

Gorsky Y, Yanky F, Sulitzeanu D (1976): Isolation from patients with breast cancer of antibodies specific for antigens associated with breast cancer and other malignant diseases. Proc Natl Acad Sci USA 73:2101–2105.

Goslin RH, O'Brien MJ, Skarin AT, Zamcheck N (1983): Immunocytochemical staining for CEA in small cell carcinoma of lung predicts clinical usefulness of the plasma assay. Cancer 52:301–306.

Gotoh YI, Sugamura K, Hinuma Y (1982): Healthy carriers of a human retrovirus, adult T-cell leukemia virus (ATLV): Demonstration by clonal culture of ATVV-carying T cells from peripheral blood. Proc Natl Acad Sci USA 79:4780–4782.

Granatek CH, Hanna MG Jr, Hersh EM, Gutterman JU, Mavligit GM, Candler EL (1976): Fetal antigens in human leukemia. Cancer Res 36:3464–3470.

Graves DT, Owen AJ, Barth RK, Tempst P, Winoto A, Fors L, Hood LE (1984): Detection of c-*sis* transcripts and synthesis of PDGF-like proteins by human osteosarcoma cells. Science 226:972–974.

Gray BN, Walker C (1983): Monitoring of patients with carcinoma of the large intestine by use of acute phase proteins and carcinoembryonic antigen. Surg Gynecol Obstet 156: 777–780.

Griffiths J (1982): The appropriate uses of prostatic acid phosphatase determination in the diagnosis of adenocarcinoma of the prostate. Ann NY Acad Sci 390:100–103.

Gronowitz JS, Hagberg H, Kallander CF, Simonsson B (1983): The use of serum deoxythymidine kinase as a prognostic marker, and in the monitoring of patients with non-Hodgkin's lymphoma. Br J Cancer 47:487–495.

Guarda LG, Ordonez NG, Smith JL, Hanssen G (1982): Immunoperoxidase localization of factor VIII in angiosarcomas. Arch Pathol Lab Med 106:515–516.

Gupta MK, Rajaraman S, Gupta SK, Hewitt CB, Deodhar SD (1981): Immunochemical measurement of serum prostatic acid phosphatase (PAP). Clinical evaluation of radioimmunoassay and counter immunoelectrophoresis. Am J Clin Pathol 76:430–436.

Gupta MK, Bolli L, Arciaga R, Tubbs R, Bukowski R, Deodhar SD (1983): Measurement of carbohydrate antigen (CA19-9) in the serum from patients with malignant and nonmalignant diseases: Comparison with CEA. Proc Am Assoc Cancer Res 23:954.

Gupta RK, Cheng LY, Leitch AM, Morton DL (1981): Characterization of tumor-associated antigen isolated from spent culture medium of a human melanoma cell line. Fed Proc 40:981.

Gusterson BA, Mitchell DP, Warburton MJ, Carter RL (1983): Epithelial markers in the diagnosis of nasopharyngeal carcinoma: An immunocytochemical study. J Clin Pathol 36:628–631.

Hagberg H, Siegbahn A (1983): Prognostic value of serum lactic dehydrogenase in non-Hodgkin's lymphoma. Scand J Haematol 31:49–56.

Hagner G (1983): Antigenic properties of human IgG kappa and IgG lambda myeloma plasma cells. Exp Hematol 11:219–225.

Haines HG, McCoy JP, Hofheinz DE, Ng AB, Nordquist SR, Leif RC (1981): Cervical carcinoma antigens in the diagnosis of human squamous cell carcinoma of the cervix. J Natl Cancer Inst 66:465–474.

Häkkinen IPT (1972): Foetal sulphoglycoprotein antigen (FSA) as a possible precursor of alimentary canal cancer. Gastroenterology 7:483–488.

Häkkinen IPT, Heinonen R, Inberg MV, Jarvi OH, Vaajalahti P, Viikari S (1980): Clinicopathological study of gastric cancers and precancerous states detected by fetal sulfoglycoprotein antigen screening. Cancer Res 40:4308–4312.

Hakomori S, Nudelman E, Levery S, Solter D, Knowles BB (1981): The hapten structure of a developmentally regulated glycolipid antigen (SSEA-1) isolated from human erythrocytes and adenocarcinoma: A preliminary note. Biochem Biophys Res Commun 100:1578–1586.

Hakomori S, Nudelman E, Levery SB, Patterson CM (1983): Human cancer-associated gangliosides defined by a monoclonal antibody (IB9) directed to sialosyl alpha 2 leads to 6 galactosyl residue: A preliminary note. Biochem Biophys Res Commun 113:791–798.

Halter SA, Dupont WD, Hartmann WH (1982): Tumor marker expression in interval breast carcinomas. Lab Invest 46:33A.

Hand PH, Nuti M, Colcher D, Schlom J (1983): Definition of antigenic heterogeneity and modulation among human mammary carcinoma cell populations using monoclonal antibodies to tumor-associated antigens. Cancer Res 43:728–735.

Hann HL, Evans AE, Siegel SE, Sather H, Hammond D, Seeger SE (1983): Serum ferritin levels as a guide to prognosis in patients with Stage IV neuroblastoma. Proc Am Soc Clin Oncol 2:C–282.

Hann HW, Kim CY, London WT, Whitford P, Blumberg BS (1982): Hepatitis B virus and primary hepatocellular carcinoma: Family studies in Korea. Int J Cancer 30:47–51.

Harach HR, Skinner M, Gibbs AR (1983): Biological markers in human lung carcinoma: An immunopathological study of six antigens. Thorax 38:937–941.

Harlozinska A, Zawadzka H, Wozniewski A, Richter R (1975): Preliminary immunologic characterization of glycoprotein antigens (CEA) of tumors of gastrointestinal tract in humans. Arch Immunol Ther Exp 23:247–255.

Harlozinska A, Lisowska E, Richter R, Albert W, Gawlikowski W, Domagala J (1980): Immunological reactivity of glycoprotein antigens from human lung cancers. Neoplasma 27:641–652.

Harper JR, Bumol TF, Reisfeld RA (1984): Characterization of monoclonal antibody 155.8 and partial characterization of its proteoglycan antigen on human melanoma cells. J Immunol 132:2096–2104.

Harris R, Viza D, Todd R, Phillips J, Sugar R, Jennison RF, Marriott G, Gleeson MH (1971): Detection of human leukaemia associated antigens in leukaemic serum and normal embryos. Nature 233:556–557.

Harvey HA, Lipton A, White D, Davidson E (1981): Glycoproteins and human cancer: II. Correlation between circulating level and disease status. Cancer 47:324–327.

Hausen A, Wachter H (1982): Pteridines in the assessment of neoplasia. J Clin Chem Clin Biochem 20:539–602.

Hayami M, Komuro A, Nozawa K, Shotake T, Ishikawa K, Yamamoto K, Ishida T, Honjo S, Hinuma Y (1984): Prevalence of antibody to adult T-cell leukemia virus-associated antigens (ATLA) in Japanese monkeys and other non-human primates. Int J Cancer 33: 179–183.

Hedin A, Carlsson L, Berglund A, Hammarstrom S (1983): A monoclonal antibody-enzyme immunoassay for serum carcinoembryonic antigen with increased specificity for carcinomas. Proc Natl Acad Sci USA 80:3470–3474.

Hehlmann R, Kufe D, Spiegelman S (1972): RNA in human leukemic cells related to the RNA of a mouse leukemia virus. Proc Natl Acad Sci USA 69:435–439.

Hehlmann R, Schetters H, Erfle V, Leilh-Mosch G (1983): Detection and biochemical characterization of antigens in human leukemic sera that cross-react with primate C-type viral proteins (Mr 30,000). Cancer Res 43:392–399.

Heisterkamp N, Stephenson JR, Groffen J, Hansen PF, de Klein A, Bartram CR, Grosveld G (1983): Localization of the c-abl oncogene adjacent to a translocation break point in chronic myelocytic leukemia. Nature 306:239–242.

Heitz PU, Kasper M, Kloppell G, Polak JM, Vaitukaitis JL (1983): Glycoprotein-hormone alpha-chain production by pancreatic endocrine tumors: A specific marker for malignancy. Immunocytochemical analysis of tumors of 155 patients. Cancer 51:277–282.

Heldman DA, Grever MR, Miser JS, Trewyn RW (1983): Relationship of urinary excretion of modified nucleosides to disease status in childhood acute lymphoblastic leukemia. J Natl Cancer Inst 71:269–273.

Hellström I, Hellström KE, Yeh MY (1981): Lymphocyte-dependent antibodies to antigen 3.1, a cell-surface antigen expressed by a subgroup of human melanomas. Int J Cancer 27:281–285.

Hellström I, Brown JP, Hellström KE (1983): Melanoma-associated antigen P97 continues to be expressed after prolonged exposure of cells to specific antibody. Int J Cancer 31: 553–555.

Helson L, Ghavimi F, Wu CJ, Fleisher M, Schwartz MK (1976): Carcinoembryonic antigen in children with neuroblastoma. J Nat Cancer Inst 57:725–726.

Henderson IC, Lokich J, Mayer R, Skarin A, Zamcheck N (1976): Carcinoembryonic antigen (CEA) levels in metastatic breast cancer: Quantitative correlation with pattern of metastases. Proc Am Assoc Cancer Res 17:202.

Hennessey PT, Hurst RE, Hemstreet GP, Cutter G (1981): Urinary glycosaminoglycan excretion as a biochemical marker in patients with bladder carcinoma. Cancer Res 41:3868–3873.

Hersey P, Honeyman M, Edwards A, Adams E, McCarthy WH (1976): Antigens on melanoma cells detected by leukocyte dependent antibody assays of human melanoma antisera. Int J Cancer 18:564–573.

Heyenga H, Morr H (1982): Diagnostic value of carcinoembryonic antigen in pleural fluid. Dtsch Med Wochenschr 107:818–821.

Heyward WL, Lanier AP, Bender TR, McMahon BJ, Kilkenny S, Paprocki TR, Kline KT, Silimperi DR, Maynard JE (1983): Early detection of primary hepatocellular carcinoma by screening for alpha-fetoprotein in high-risk families. A case-report. Lancet 2: 1161–1162.

Higgins PJ, Friedman E, Lipkin M, Hertz R, Attiyeh F (1981): Transformation associated fetal antigens in human premalignant colonic epithelial cells. Gastroenterology 80:1174.

Higgins PJ, Correa P, Cuello C, Kipkin M (1983a): Fetal antigens in precursor stages of gastric cancer. Proc Am Assoc Cancer Res 24:506.

Higgins PJ, Friedman E, Lipkin M, Hertz R, Attiyeh F, Stonehill EH (1983b): Expression of gastric-associated antigens by human premalignant and malignant colonic epithelial cells. Oncology 40:26–30.

Hill SA, Hunt WE (1982): CEA in brain tumor cyst fluids. Surg Form 33:519–521.

Hino O, Kitagawa T, Koike K, Kohayashi M, Hara M, Mori W, Nakashima T, Hattori N, Sagano H (1984): Detection of hepatitis B virus DNA in hepatocellular carcinomas in Japan. Hepatology 4:90–95.

Hinuma Y (1983): Adult T-cell leukemia virus—Introduction. Gan To Kagaku Ryoho 10: 659–662.

Hirohashi S, Shimosato Y, Ino Y, Kishi K, Ohkura H, Mukojima T (1983): Distribution of alpha-fetoprotein and immunoreactive carcinoembryonic antigen in human hepatocellular carcinoma and hepatoblastoma. Jpn J Clin Oncol 13:37–44.

Hirshaut Y, Katopodis N, Pinola C, Spector K, Godbold J, Schottenfeld D, Stock CC (1983): LSA test results in children with sarcoma and their families—LSA values have prognostic significance. Proc Am Assoc Cancer Res 23:504.

Hishiki S, Sakaguchi S, Kanno T (1984): Clinical significance of acidic pI isoenzyme of ribonuclease in human serum. Clin Chim Acta 136:155–164.

Hitchcock MH, Hollinshead AC, Chretien P, Rizzoli HV (1979): Soluble membrane antigens of brain tumors: I. Controlled testing for cell-mediated immune response in a long surviving glioblastoma multiforme patient. Cancer 40:660–666.

Ho JH, Lau WH, Kwan HG, Chan CL, Au GH, Saw D (1982): Immunology and diagnosis of nasopharyngeal carcinoma. Excerpta Med Int Congr Ser 571:389–397.

Hobbs JR, Knapp ML, Branfoot AC (1980): Pancreatic oncofetal antigen (POA): Its frequency and localization. Oncodev Biol Med 1:37–48.

Hockey MS, Stokes HJ, Thompson H, Woodhouse CS, MacDonald F, Fielding JW, Ford CH (1984): Carcinoembryonic antigen (CEA) expression and heterogeneity in primary and autologous metastatic gastric tumors demonstrated by a monoclonal antibody. Br J Cancer 49:129–133.

Hofstadter F, Jakse G (1982): The significance of ABH-antigens and CEA in the prognosis of urothelial tumors. Wien Klin Wochenschr 94:366–368.

Hokin K, Abe H, Aida T, Mabuchi S, Tsuru M, Nakamura N (1983): Primary intracranial germ cell tumor with abnormal high value of alpha fetoprotein after the radiation therapy. No Shinkei Geka 11:217–221.

Holden S, Bernard O, Artzt K, Whitmoer WF, Bennett D (1977): Human and mouse embryonal carcinoma cells in culture share an embryonic antigen (F9). Nature 270: 518–520.

Holder WD, Wells SA (1983): Antibody reacting with the murine mammary tumor virus in the serum of patients with breast carcinoma: A possible serological detection method for breast carcinoma. Cancer Res 43:239–244.

Hollinshead A, Miller H, Tanner K, Lee O, Klausia J (1979): Soluble cell membrane antigens associated with bladder cancer. Cancer Immunol Immunother 5:93–103.

Hollinshead AC (1975): Analysis of soluble melanoma cell membrane antigens in metastatic cells of various organs and further studies of antigens present in primary melanoma. Cancer 36:1282–1288.

Hollinshead AC, Jaffurs WT, Alpert LK, Harris JE, Herberman RB (1974): Isolation and identification of soluble skin-reactive membrane antigens of malignant and normal human breast cells. Cancer Res 34:2961–2968.

Hollinshead AC, Sega E, Stewart THM, Ricci C, Mineo TC (1975): Comparison of lung cancer antigens. Tumori 61:125–128.

Holton OD, Lovins RE, Fudenberg HH (1980): Antibody affinity isolation and electrophoretic characterization of a plasma membrane antigen associated with human breast cancer. Fed Proc 39:352.

Hook RR Jr, Hamby CV, Millikan LE, Berkelhammer J, Stills HF Jr, Oxenhandler RW (1983): Cell-mediated immune reactivity of Sinclair melanoma-bearing swine to 3MKCl extracts of swine and human melanoma. Int J Cancer 31:633–637.

Hopkins SC, Nissenkorn I, Palmieri GM, Ikard M, Moinuddin M, Soloway MS (1983): Serial spot hydroxyproline/creatinine ratios in metastatic prostatic cancer. J Urol 129:319–323.

Horgan IE (1982): Total and lipid-bound sialic acid levels in sera from patients with cancer. Clin Chim Acta 118:327–331.

Horie Y, Gomyoda M, Kishimoto Y, Ueki J, Ikeda F, Murawaki Y, Kawamura M, Hirayma C (1984): Plasma carcinoembryonic antigen and acinar cell carcinoma of the pancreas. Cancer 53:1137–1142.

Horn U, Beal SL, Walach N, Lubich WP, Spigel L, Marton LJ (1982): Further evidence for the use of polyamines as biochemical markers for malignant tumors. Cancer Res 42: 3248–3251.

Hua DT, Princler GL, Braatz JA (1984): Comparison of an enzyme-linked immunosorbent assay (ELISA) and a radioimmunoassay (RIA) for measuring serum levels of a lung tumor-associated antigen (LTA). Fed Proc 43:1750.

Huber PR, Geyer E, Kung W, Matter A, Torhorst J, Eppenberger U (1978): Retinoic acid-binding protein in human breast cancer and dysplasia. J Natl Cancer Inst 61:1375–1378.

Huber PR, Zaugg T, Linder E, Hagmaier V, Rutishauser G (1982): Creatine kinase isoenzyme (CK-BB) in combination with prostatic acid phosphatase measured by RIA in the diagnosis of prostatic cancer.. Urol Res 10:75–80.

Huber PR, Rist M, Hering F, Biedermann C, Rutishauser G (1983): Tissue polypeptide antigen (TPA) and prostatic acid phosphatase in serum of prostatic cancer patients. Urol Res 11:223–226.

Huhtala ML, Kahanpaa K, Seppala M, Halila H, Stenman UH (1983): Excretion of a tumor-associated trypsin inhibitor (TATI) in urine of patients with gynecological malignancy. Int J Cancer 31:711–714.

Hull JC, Carlo JR, DeFazio SR, Monaco AP, Gozzo JJ (1984): Immunocytochemical identification of a tumor-associated antigen in carcinoma of the urinary bladder. Fed Proc 43:1420.

Humphrey LJ, Estes NC, Morse PA, Jewell WR, Boudet RA, Hudson MJK, Tsolakidis PG, Mantz FA (1974): Serum antibody in patients with breast disease: Correlation with histopathology. Ann Surg 180:124–128.

Hurlimann J, Dayal R (1978): Antigen of a human breast carcinoma cell line (BT20). I. Synthesis of serum proteins, membrane-associated antigens, and oncofetal-associated antigens. J Natl Cancer Inst 61:677–685.

Huseby NE, Eide TJ (1983): Variant gamma-glutamyltransferases in colorectral carcinomas. Clin Chim Acta 135:301–307.

Huth JF, Gupta RK, Morton DL (1981): Development of an enzyme immunoassay to detect and quantitate tumor-associated antigens in the urine of sarcoma patients. Cancer 47: 2856–2861.

Huth JF, Gupta RK, Eilber FR, Morton DL (1984): A prospective postoperative evaluation of urinary tumor-associated antigens in sarcoma patients. Correlation with disease recurrence. Cancer 53:1306–1310.

Ibrahim AN, Rawlins D, Abdelal A, Azhar A, Swaminathan V, Mansour K, Nahmias A (1980): Tumor-associated antigens in lung cancer tissues and in sera of tumor-bearing patients. Cell Mol Biol 26:327–333.

Iizuka S, Taniguchi N, Makita A (1984): Enzyme-linked immunosorbent assay for human manganese-containing superoxide dismutase and its content in lung cancer. J Natl Cancer Inst 72:1043–1049.

Imal K, Ng AK, Ferrone S (1981): Characterization of monoclonal antibodies to human melanoma-associated antigens. J Natl Cancer Inst 66:489–496.

Imam A, Taylor CE, Tokes ZA (1983): Human monoclonal antibodies: Their use for investigating the antigenic heterogeneity of malignant breast epithelial cells. Proc Am Assoc Cancer Res 23:866.

Imamura N, Takahashi T, Lloyd KO, Lewis JL, Old LJ (1978): Analysis of human ovarian tumor antigens using heterologous antisera: Detection of new antigenic systems. Int J Cancer 21:570–577.

Inaba N, Ishige H, Ijichi M, Satoh N, Ohkawa R, Sekiya S, Shirotake S, Takamizawa H, Renk T, Bohn H (1982): Immunohistochemical detection of pregnancy-specific protein (SPI) and placenta-specific tissue proteins (PP5,PP10,PP11, and PP12) in ovarian adenocarcinomas. Oncodev Biol Med 3:379–389.

Iqbai MP, Rothenberg SP (1981): A nonfunctional protein in human leukemia cells reacts with antiserum to dihydrofolate reductase from L 1210 leukemia cells. Life Sci 29:689–696.

Irie RF, Irie K, Morton DL (1976): A membrane antigen common to human cancer and fetal brain tissues. Cancer Res 36:3510–3517.

Irie RF, Jones PC, Morton DL, Sidell N (1981): In vitro production of human antibody to a tumour-associated foetal antigen. Br J Cancer 44:262–266.

Ishiguro Y, Kato K, Shimizu A, Ito T, Nagaya M (1982): High levels of immunoreactive nervous system-specific enolase sera of patients with neuroblastoma. Clin Chim Acta 121:173–180.

Ishii M (1978): A new carcinoembryonic protein characterized by basic property. Scand J Immunol 8:611–620.

Ishii J, Kanda Y (1980): Isolation and physicochemical and immunological studies of basic fetoprotein. Proc 39th Annu Meet Jpn Cancer Assoc, Tokyo, p 367.

Ishii Y, Goldhofer W, Mavligit GM (1980): Surface antigenic characteristics of human melanoma cells defined by xenoantiserum against papain-solubilized melanoma-associated antigens. Gan 71:811–888.

Jacob F (1977): Mouse teratocarcinoma and embryonic antigens. Immunol Rev 33:4–32.

Jacobs C, Rubsamen H (1983): Expression of pp60c-src protein kinase in adult and fetal human tissue: High activities in some sarcomas and mammary carcinomas. Cancer Res 43:1696–1702.

Jakse G, Rauschmeier H, Rosmanith P, Hofstadter F (1983): Determination of carcinoembryonic antigen in tissue, serum and urine in patients with transitional cell carcinoma of the urinary bladder. Urol Int 38:121–125.

Jalanko H, Kuusela P, Roberts P, Sipponeh P, Haglund CA, Makela O (1984): Comparison of a new tumour marker CA19-9, with alpha-fetoprotein and carcinoembryonic antigen in patients with upper gastrointestinal diseases. J Clin Pathol 37:218–222.

Javadpour N (1983): Multiple biochemical tumor markers in seminoma. A double-blind study. Cancer 52:887–889.

Javadpour N, Bergman S (1978): Recent advances in testicular cancer. Curr Probl Surg 15:1–64.

Jenson AB, Lancaster WD, Hartmann DP, Shaffer EL (1982a): Frequency and distribution of papilloma virus structural antigens in verrucae, multiple papillomas, and condylomata of the oral cavity. Am J Pathol 107:212–218.

Jenson AB, Sommer S, Payling-Wright C, Pass F, Link CC, Lancaster WD (1982b): Human papillomavirus. Frequency and distribution in plantar and common warts. Lab Invest 47:491–497.

Jones PC, Sze LL, Liu PY, Morton DL, Irie RF (1981): Prolonged survival for melanoma patients with elevated IgM antibody to oncofetal antigen. J Natl Cancer Inst 66:249–254.

Jothy S, Brenner B, Fuks A, Shuster J (1982): Immunohistologic characterization of a monoclonal antibody directed against squamous cell carcinoma of the lung. Lab Invest 46:43A.

Jozwiak W, Koscielak J (1980): Occurrence of lactosylsphingosine-reactive antibodies in sera of cancer patients. Acta Haematol Pol 11:173–179.

Jozwiak W, Koscielak J (1982): Lactosylsphingosine-reactive antibody and CEA in patients with colorectal cancer. Eur J Cancer Clin Oncol 18:617–621.

Kabawat SE, Bast RC Jr, Bhan AK, Welch WR, Knapp RC, Colvin RB (1983): Tissue distribution of a coelomic-epithelium-related antigen recognized by the monoclonal antibody OC125. Int J Gynecol Pathol 2:375–378.

Kabisch H, Thiele HG, Winkler K, Landbeck G (1978): Partial molecular characterization of an antigenic structure associated to cells of common acute lymphocytic leukemia (ALL). Clin Exp Immunol 32:399–404.

Kalashnikov VV, Borisenko SA, Tatarinov YS, (1976): Immunochemical identification of a new embryonic antigen in ovarian tumor tissue. Bull Exp Biol Med 81:900–902.

Kalashnikov VV, Chekhonin VP, Tatarinov YS (1983): Interspecies embryonic antigens in the blood serum of cancer patients. Vopr Onkol 29:24–29.

Kalyanaraman VS, Sarngadharan MG, Poiesz B, Ruscetti FW, Gallo RC (1981): Immunological properties of a type C retrovirus isolated from cultured human T-lymphoma cells and comparison to other mammalian retroviruses. J Virol 38:906–915.

Kalyanaraman VS, Sarngadharan MG, Robert-Guroff M, Miyoshi I, Blayney D, Golde D, Gallo RC (1982): A new subtype of human T-cell leukemia virus (HTLV-II) associated with a T-cell variant of hairy cell leukemia. Science 218:571–573.

Kamiyama M, Hashim GA, Kyriakidis G, Fitzpatrick HF (1980): A tumor-associated antigen isolated from human breast adenocarcinoma. Clin Immunol Immunopathol 16:151–165.

Kariniemi, AL, Forsman L, Wahlstrom T, Vesterinen E, Andersson C (1984): Expression of differentiation antigens in mammary and extramammary Paget's disease. Br J Dermatol 110:203–210.

Kasai M, Saxton RE, Holmes EC, Burk MW, Morton DL (1981): Membrane antigens detected on human lung carcinoma cells by hybridoma monoclonal antibody. J Surg Res 30: 403–408.

Kaszurbowski PA, Terasaki PI, Chia DS, Kukes GD, Hardiwidjaja SI, Cicciarelli JC (1984): A cytotoxic monoclonal antibody to colon adenocarcinoma. Cancer Res 44:1194–1199.

Katano M, Sidell N, Irie RF (1983): Human monoclonal antibody to a neuroectodermal tumor antigen (OFA-I-2). Ann NY Acad Sci 417:427–434.

Katayama I, Shibuya A, Niikawa K, Nanba K, Kogat T, Toyama K (1984): Demonstration of p35 in hairy cell leukemia of Japanese patients. Cancer 53:2111–2114.

Kato H, Morioka H, Aramaki S, Torigoe T (1979): Radioimmunoassay for tumor-antigen of human cervical squamous cell carcinoma. Cell Mol Biol 25:51–56.

Kato H, Morioka H, Aramaki S, Tamai K, Torigoe T (1983): Prognostic significance of the tumor antigen TA-4 in squamous cell carcinoma of the uterine cervix. Am J Obstet Gynecol 145:350–354.

Katopodis N, Hirshaut Y, Stock CC (1983): Influence of processing interval on LSA test sensitivity. Proc Am Assoc Cancer Res 23:298.

Kaufman RH, Dreesman GR, Burek J, Korhonen MO, Matson DO, Melnick JL, Powell KL, Purifoy DJM, Courtney RJ, Adam E (1981): Herpesvirus-induced antigens in squamous-cell carcinoma in situ of the vulva. N Engl J Med 305:483–488.

Kawano V (1983): Localization of hepatitis B surface antigen in hepatocellular carcinoma. Acta Pathol Jpn 33:1087–1093.

Kawata M, Higaki K, Sekiya S, Takamizawa H, Muramatsu T, Okumura K (1983): Antibodies to large glycopeptide in sera from patients with ovarian germ cell tumours. Clin Exp Immunol 51:401–406.

Kehayov I, Botev B, Vulchanov V, Kyurkchiev S (1976): Demonstration of a phase (stage)-specific embryonic brain antigen in human meningioma. Int J Cancer 18:587–592.

Kehayov IR (1976): Tumour-associated water soluble antigen(s) in human glioblastoma demonstrated by immunodiffusion and immunoelectrophoresis. Ann Immunol 127:703–716.

Kehayov IR, Vetzka PF, Ivanov GL, Kyurkchiev SD (1977): Purification of human meningioma-associated antigen by gel-chromatography. Dokl Bulg Akad Nauk 30:621–624.

Kehayov IR, Kyurkchiev SD, Botev BA, Vetzka PF (1979): An onco-fetal antigen in human medulloblastoma. C R Acad Bulg Sci 32:217–220.

Kelly B, Levy JG (1977): Evidence for a common tumour-associated antigen in extracts of human bronchogenic carcinoma. Br J Cancer 35:828–833.

Kelly BS, Levy JG (1980): Tumour-associated antigens in lung cancer: The possibility for a serologic assay. Can Med Assoc J 122:1020–1023.

Kelsey DE, Busch RK, Busch H (1981): An enzyme immunoassay for the detection of human tumor nucleolar antigens. Cancer Lett 12:295–303.

Kempner DH, Jay MR, Stevens RH (1979): Human lung tumor-associated antigens of 32,000 daltons molecular weight. J Natl Cancer Inst 63:1121–1129.

Kennett RH, Gilbert F (1979): Hybrid myelomas producing antibodies against a human neuroblastoma antigen present on fetal brain. Science 203:1120–1121.

Kerney SE, Montague PM, Chertien PB, Nicholson JM, Ekel TM, Hearing VJ (1977): Intracellular localization of tumor-associated antigens in murine and human malignant melanoma. Cancer Res 37:1519–1524.

Keydar I, Ohno T, Nayak R, Sweet R, Simon F, Weiss F, Karby S, Mesa-Tejada R, Spiegelman S (1984): Properties of retrovirus-like particles produced by a human breast carcinoma cell line: Immunological relationship with mouse mammary tumor virus proteins. Proc Natl Acad Sci USA 81:4188–4192.

Khan A, Grammer S, Chang D, Hill NO, Miller J (1983): Mouse monoclonal antibody (WI-MN-1) against malignant melanoma. Cancer Res 43:5868–5872.

Khan O, Hensley CN, Williams G (1982): Prostacyclin in prostatic cancer: A better marker than bone scan or serum acid phosphatase? Br J Urol 54:26–31.

Khoo SK, Hill R, Daunter B, Mackay EV (1982): Carcinoembryonic antigen in ovarian cancer: Correlation of concentrations in tumour tissue, cyst fluid, ascitic fluid, and peripheral blood. Aust NZ Obstet Gynecol 22:65–70.

Khosravi M, Dent PB, Liao SK (1983): Structural and biosynthetic studies of a human melanoma specific oncofetal antigen defined by the monoclonal antibody 140, 240. Proc Am Assoc Cancer Res 23:860.

Kiang DT, Greenberg LJ (1983): CEA in designing chemotherapy for advanced breast cancers. Proc Am Soc Clin Oncol 2:C-406.

Kikuchi Y, Kizawa I, Koyama E, Kato K (1984): Significance of serum tumor markers in patients with carcinoma of the ovary. Obstet Gynecol 63:561–566.

Kim H, Pangalis GA, Payne BC, Kadin ME, Rappaport H (1982): Ultrastructural identification of neoplastic histiocytes-monocytes. An application of a newly developed cytochemical technique. Am J Pathol 106:204–223.

Kindblom LG, Jacobson GK, Jacobsen M (1982): Immunohistochemical investigations of tumor of supposed fibroblastic-histiocytic origin. Hum Pathol 13:834–840.

Kingsnorth AN, Wallace HM, Bundred NJ, Dixon JM (1984): Polyamines in breast cancer. Br J Surg 71:532–536.

Kioussis D, Eiferman F, van de Riju P, Gorin MB, Ingram RS, Tilghman SM (1981): The evolution of α-fetoprotein and albumin. II. The structures of the α-fetoprotein and albumin genes in the mouse. J Biol Chem 256:1960–1967.

Kirsch J, Oehr P, Winkler C (1983): Localization of tissue polypeptide antigen in interphase HeLa cells by immunofluorescence microscopy. Tumor Diagn Ther 4:222–224.

Kistler GS, Sonnabend W (1974): Antikörper gegen ein fetorenales Antigen in Hepatitis-B-Patienten, Trägern von Nierentumoren und gesunden Individuen. Schweiz Med Wochenschr 104:485–497.

Kivela T, Tarkkanen A (1983): Carcinoembryonic antigen in retinoblastoma. An immunohistochemical study. Graefes Arch Clin Exp Ophthalmol 221:8–11.

Kizawa I, Kikuchi Y, Kato K (1983): Diagnostic value of biochemical tumor markers in serum of patients with cancer of the ovary. Nippon Sanka Fujinka Gakkai Zasshi 35:251–258.

Kjaer M, Fischerman K (1976): Carcinoembryonic antigen (CEA): A prospective clinical trial in patients with gastrointestinal cancer. Scand J Gastroenterol 11:99–106.

Kjorstad KE, Orjasester H (1982): The prognostic value of CEA determiniations in the plasma of patients with squamous cell cancer of the cervix. Cancer 50:283–287.

Klavins JV (1981): Tumor markers of pancreatic carcinoma. Cancer 47:1597–1601.

Klavins JV (1982a): Definition and classification of tumor markers. Ann Clin Lab Sci 12: 331–332.

Klavins JV (1982b): Classification of biochemical tumor markers. Cancer Det Prev 5:88.

Klavins JV (1983): Gastrointestinal tumor markers, other than carcinoembryonic antigen, and alpha fetal protein. In Nieburgs HE, Birkmayer GD, Klavins JV (eds): "Human Tumor Markers: Biological Basis and Clinical Relevance." New York: Alan R. Liss, pp 131–136.

Klavins JV, Cho YT (1983): Preliminary studies in comparing carcinoembryonic antigen (CEA) with tissue polypeptide antigen (TPA). Cancer Det Prev 6:582.

Klavins JV, Mesa-Tejada R, Weiss M (1971): Human carcinoma antigens cross reacting with anti-embryonic antibodies. Nature New Biol 234:153–154.

Klavins JV, Berkman JI, Mesa-Tejada R, Weiss M, Krauss E (1974a): Embryonic proteins in malignant neoplasms. In Bucalossi P, Veronesi U, Cascinella N (eds): "Proc XI Int Cancer Congress, Vol 1. Cell Biology and Tumor Immunology." Amsterdam: Excerpta Medica, pp 200–207.

Klavins JV, Weiss M, Mesa-Tejada R, Fierer JA, Berkman JI (1974b): Recently defined oncofetal antigens and their potential application in clinical medicine. Ann Clin Lab Sci 4: 139–144.

Klavins JV, Shapiro SH, Wessely Z, Berkman JI (1980): RNA virus associated antigen in human placenta. Ann Clin Lab Sci 10:137–142.

Klein G, Steiner M, Wiener F, Klein E (1974): Human leukemia-associated anti-nuclear reactivity. Proc Natl Acad Sci USA 71:685–689.

Klein G, Manneborg-Sandlund A, Ehlin-Henriksson B, Godal T, Wiels J, Tursz T (1983): Expression of the BLA antigen, defined by the monoclonal 38.13 antibody, on Burkitt lymphoma lines, lymphoblastoid cell lines, their hybrids and other B-cell lymphomas and leukemias. Int J Cancer 31:535–542.

Knapp ML (1981): Partial characterization of an oncofetal pancreatic antigen. Ann Clin Biochem 18:131–142.

Knauf S, Urbach GI (1981): Identification, purification, and radioimmunoassay of NB70K, a human ovarian tumor-associated antigen. Cancer Res 41:1351–1357.

Knauf S, Taillon-Miller P, Helmkamp BF, Bonfiglio TA, Beecham JB (1984): Selectivity for ovarian cancer of an improved serum radioimmunoassay for human ovarian tumor-associated antigen NB/70K. Gynecol Oncol 17:349–355.

Knowles BB, Rappaport J, Solter D (1982): Murine embryonic antigen (SSEA-1) is expressed on human cells and structurally related human blood group antigen I is expressed on mouse embryos. Dev Biol 93:54–58.

Koestler TP, Papsidero LD, Nemoto T, Chu TM (1981): Detection of breast tissue-associated antigen by antiserum to Raji cell-bound circulating immune complexes of human breast cancer. Cancer Res 41:2900–2907.

Koistinen R, Heikinheim M, Rutanen E-M, Stenman U-H, Lee JN, Seppala M (1981): Concanavalin A binding of pregnancy-specific beta-1-glycoprotein in normal pregnancy and trophoblastic disease. Oncodev Biol Med 2:179–182.

Koprowki H, Herlyn M, Steplewski Z (1981): Specific antigen in serum of patients with colon carcinomas. Science 212:53–55.

Korosteleva TA, Melnikov RA, Belokhvostova AT (1976): Antigen containing the tryptophane metabolite 3-oxyanthranilic acid in blood serum of patients with stomach tumors. Vopr Onkol 22:22–26.

Korosteleva VS (1957): Similarities and differences of specific antigens of cancer in man. Oncology 44:987–993.

Kosaki T, Ikoda T, Kotani Y, Nakagawa S, Saka T (1958): A new phospholipid, malignolipin, in human malignant tumors. Science 127:1176–1177.

Kouttab NM, Bowen JM, Dmochowski L, Von Eschenbach A, Bracken RB, Johnson D (1978): Search for type C virus-like information in normal, benign and malignant human prostatic tissue. Tex J Science 30:139–148.

Kozielski J (1982): Carcinoembryonic antigen (CEA), alpha-fetoprotein and chorion gonadotropin (HCG) in patients with primary carcinoma of the lung. Eur J Respir Dis 63:112.

Krauss S, Macy S, Ichiki AT (1981): A study of immunoreactive calcitonin (CT), adrenocorticotropic hormone (ACTH) and carcinoembryonic antigen (CEA) in lung cancer and other malignancies. Cancer 47:2485–2492.

Krieger G, Wander HE, Prangen M, Bandlow G, Beyer JH, Nagel GA (1983): Determination of the carcinoembryonic antigen (CEA) for predicting the success of therapy in metastatic breast cancer. Dtsch Med Wochenschr 108:610–614.

Krueger RG, Staneck LD, Boehlecke M (1976): Tumor-associated antigens in human myeloma. J Natl Cancer Inst 56:711–715.

Kufe D, Hehlmann R, Spiegelman S (1972): Human sarcomas contain RNA related to the RNA of mouse leukemia virus. Science 175:182–185.

Kufe DW, Peters WP, Spiegelman S (1973a): Unique nuclear DNA sequences in the involved tissues of Hodgkin's and Burkitt's lymphomas. Proc Natl Acad Sci USA 70:3810–3814.

Kufe D, Magrath JT, Ziegler JL, Spiegelman S (1973b): Burkitt's tumors contain particles encapsulating RNA-instructed DNA polymerase and high molecular weight virus. Proc Natl Acad Sci USA 70:737–741.

Kufe D, Hehlmann R, Spiegelmann S (1973c): RNA related to that of a murine leukemia virus in Burkitt's tumors and nasopharyngeal carcinomas. Proc Natl Acad Sci USA 70: 5–9.

Kufe DW, Nadler L, Sargent L, Shapiro H, Hand P, Austin F, Colcher D, Schlom J (1983): Biological behavior of human breast carcinoma-associated antigens expressed during cellular proliferation. Cancer Res 43:851–857.

Kuhajda FP, Mann RB (1984): Adenoid cystic carcinoma of the prostate. A case report with immunoperoxidase staining for prostate-specific acid phosphatase and prostate-specific antigen. Am J Clin Pathol 81:257–260.

Kuhajda FP, Taxy JB (1983): Oncofetal antigens in sacrococcygeal teratomas. Arch Pathol Lab Med 107:239–242.

Kumar S, Costello CB, Glashan RW, Björklund B (1981): The clinical significance of tissue polypeptide antigen (TPA) in the urine of bladder cancer patient. Br J Urol 53:573–581.

Kuntz DL, Archer SJ (1979): Extraction and identification of a human pancreatic-tumor associated antigen. Oncology 36:134–138.

Kuo T, Rosai J, Tillack TW (1973): Isolation of a tumor associated antigen from human breast carcinoma and its relationship to CEA. Fed Proc 32:859.

Kuriyama M, Wang MC, Papsidero LD, Shimano T, Valenzuela L, Murphy GP, Chu TM (1980): Immunologic detection of a prostate specific antigen in human prostate cancer. Proc Am Assoc Cancer Res 21:207.

Kurman RJ, Scardino P, McIntire KR, Waldmann RA, Javadpour N (1977): Cellular localization of alpha-fetoprotein and human chorionic gonadotropin in germ cell tumors of the testis using an indirect immunoperoxidase technique: A new approach to classification utilizing tumor markers. Cancer 40:2136–2151.

Kurman RJ, Shah KH, Lancaster WD, Jenson AB (1981): Immunoperoxidase localization of papillomavirus antigens in cervical dysplasia and vulvar condylomas, Am J Obstet Gyncol 140:931–935.

Kurman RJ, Sanz LE, Jenson AB, Perry S, Lancaster WD (1982): Papillomavirus infection of the cervix. I. Correlation of histology with viral structural antigens and DNA sequences. Int J Gynecol Pathol 1:17–28.

Kurman RJ, Jenson AB, Lancaster WD (1983): Papillomavirus infection of the cervix. II Relationship to intraepithelial neoplasia based on the presence of specific viral structural proteins. Am J Surg Pathol 7:39–52.

Kurth R, Lower J, Lower R, Wernicke D, Frank H (1981): Human teratocarcinomas produce unique oncovirus-like particle. In "RNA Tumor Viruses, May 20–24, 1981." Cold Spring Harbor, New York: Cold Spring Harbor Laboratory.

Kuusela P, Jalanko H, Roberts P, Sipponen P, Mecklin JP, Pitkanen R, Makela O (1984): Comparison of CA19-9 and carcinoembryonic antigen (CEA) levels in the serum of patients with colorectal diseases. Br J Cancer 49:135–139.

Kwee WS, Veldhuizen RW, Golding RP, Mullink H, Stam J, Donner R, Boon ME (1982): Histologic distinction between malignant mesothelioma, benign pleural lesion and carcinoma metastasis. Evaluation of the application of morphometry combined with histochemistry and immunostaining. Virchows Arch 397:287–299.

Lancaster WD, Jenson AB (1981): Evidence for papillomavirus genus-specific antigens and DNA in laryngeal papilloma. Intervirology 15:204–211.

Lane MA, Sainten A, Cooper GM (1981): Activation of related transforming genes in mouse and human mammary carcinomas. In "RNA Tumor Viruses, May 20–24, 1981." Cold Spring Harbor, New York: Cold Spring Harbor Laboratory.

Lange PH, Vogelzang NJ, Goldman A, Kennedy BJ, Fraley EE (1982a): Marker half-life analysis as a prognostic tool in testicular cancer. J Urol 128:708–711.

Lange PH, Versella RL, Millan JL, Stigbrand T, Ruoslahti E, Fishman WH (1982b): The Clinical importance of placental alkaline phosphatase as a tumor marker in seminoma. In "77th Annual Meeting of the American Urological Association, May 16–20, 1982, Kansas City, Missouri." American Urological Association.

Larson SM, Brown JP, Wright PW, Carrasquillo JA, Hellström I, Hellström KE (1983): Imaging of melanoma with I-131-labeled monoclonal antibodies. J Nucl Med 24:123–129.

Laurent R, Kienzler JL, Croissant O, Orth G (1982): Two anatomoclinical types of warts with plantar localization: Specific cytopathogenic effects of papillomavirus type 1 (HPV-1) and type 2 (HPV-2). Arch Dermatol Res 274:101–111.

Lawrence EC, Broder S, Jaffe ES, Braylan RC, Dobbins WO, Young RC, Waldmann TA (1978): Evaluation of a lymphoma with helper T-cell characteristics in Sézary's syndrome. Blood 52:481–492.

Lazarus LH, DiAugustine RP, Jahnke GD, Hernandez O (1983): Physalaemin: An amphibian tachykinin in human lung small-cell carcinoma. Science 219:79–81.

Leader M, Jass JR (1984): Increased α-fetoprotein concentration in association with ileal adenocarcinoma complicating Crohn's disease. J Clin Pathol 37:293–297.

Lee AK, DeLellis RA, Rosen PP, Herbert-Stanton T, Tallberg K, Garcia C, Wolfe HJ (1984): Alpha-lactalbumin as an immunohistochemical marker for metastatic breast carcinomas. Am J Surg Pathol 8:93–100.

Lee JN, Wahlstrom T, Ouyang PC, Chen TY, Seppala M (1981): Immunohistochemical evidence for prolactin in trophoblastic tumors. Gynecol Oncol 11:299–303.

Lee W-H, Murphree AL, Benedict WF (1984): Expression and amplification of the N-myc gene in primary retinoblastoma. Nature 309:458–460.

Lee YT (1983): Serial tests of carcinoembryonic antigen in patients with breast cancer. Am J Clin Oncol 6:287–293.

Lehmann FG (1975): Immunological relationship between human placental and intestinal alkaline phosphatase. Clin Chim Acta 65:257–269.

Lennert K (1978): Malignant lymphomas other than Hodgkin's disease. In collaboration with H. Mohri, H. Stein, E. Kaiserling, HK Muller-Hermelink. In: "Handbuch der Speziellen Pathologischen Anatomie und Histologie." Berlin: Springer Verlag.

Leong SPL, Cooperband SR, Sutherland CM, Krementz ET, Deckers PJ (1978): Detection of human melanoma antigens in cell-free supernatants. J Surg Res 24:245–252.

Lerner MP, Anglin JH, Nordquist RE (1978): Cell-surface antigens from human breast tumor cells. J Natl Cancer Inst 60:39–44.

Leroux D, Pourny C, Desoize B, Jardiller JC (1978): Phosphohexose isomerase as an index of breast cancer: Evolution under chemotherapy. LARC Med Sci (Cancer) 6:68.

Leung JP, Nelson-Rees WA, Moore GE, Cailleau R, Edgington TS (1981): Characteristics of membrane and cytosol forms of the mammary tumor glycoprotein molecule MTGP in human breast carcinoma cell cultures and tumors. Int J Cancer 28:35–42.

Lewi H, Blumgart LH, Carter DC, Gillis CR, Hole D, Ratcliffe JG, Wood CB, McArdle CS (1984): Pre-operative carcinembryomic antigen and survival in patients with colorectal cancer. Br J Surg 71:206–208.

Lewis MG, Avis PJG, Phillips TM, Sheikh KMA (1973): Tumor-associated antigens in human malignant melanoma. Yale J Biol Med 46:661-668.

Liao S-K, Kwong PC, Dent PB (1980): Interferon enhances the expression of melanoma-associated antigens and beta-2 microglobulin in cultured human melanoma cells. Proc Am Assoc Cancer Res 21:205.

Liao S-K, Clarke BJ, Kwong PC, Brickenden A, Gallie BL, Dent PB (1981): Common neuroectodermal antigens on human melanoma, neuroblastoma, retinoblastoma, glioblastoma and fetal brain revealed by hybridoma antibodies raised against melanoma cells. Eur J Immunol 11:450–454.

Liao S-K, Clarke BJ, Khosravi M, Kwong PC, Brickenden A, Dent PB (1982): Human melanoma-specific oncofetal antigen defined by a mouse monoclonal antibody. Int J Cancer 30:573–580.

Liao S-K, Kwong PC, Khosravi M, Clarke BJ, Dent PB (1983): 140.72: A mouse monoclonal antibody recognizing human melanoma/carcinoma crossreacting antigen(s) associated with carcinoembryonic antigen. Proc Am Assoc Cancer Res 23:918.

Lichtiger B, Trujillo JM, Burk KH, Drewinko B (1976): Identification and subcellular localization of a sarcoma-associated antigen(s) in a human cell line. Cancer 37:1788–1799.

Liebman HA, Furie BC, Tong MJ, Blanchard RA, Lo KJ, Lee SD, Coleman MS, Furie B (1984): Des-gamma-carboxyl (abnormal) prothrombin as a serum marker of primary hepatocellular carcinoma. N Engl J Med 310:1427–1431.

Lindemalm C, Biberfeld P, Bjorkholm M, Henle G, Henle W, Holm G, Johansson B, Klein G, Mellstedt H (1983): Epstein-Barr virus-associated antibody pattern in unrelated non-Hodgkin lymphoma patients. Relationship to clinical variables and lymphocyte functions. Int J Cancer 32:675–682.

Lindholm L, Holmgren J, Svennerholm L, Freedman PE, Nilsson D, Persson B, Myrvol H, Lagergard T (1983): Monoclonal antibodies against gastrointestinal tumour-associated antigens isolated as monosialogangliosides. Int Arch Allergy Appl Immunol 71:178–181.

Linkesch W, Ludwig H (1982): Serum ferritin and beta-2-microglobulin in multiple myeloma. Acta Med Aust 9:227–231.

Little CD, Nau MM, Carney DN, Gazdar AF, Minna JD (1983): Amplification and expression of the c-myc oncogene in human lung cancer cell lines. Nature 306:194–196.

Lloyd JM, O'Dowd T, Driver M, Deh Tee (1984): Demonstration of an epitope of the transferrin receptor in human cervical epithelium—A potentially useful cell marker. J Clin Pathol 37:131–135.

Lloyd RV, Rosen PP, Sarkar NH, Jimenez D, Kinne DW, Menendez-Botet C, Schwartz MK (1983): Murine mammary tumor virus related antigen in human male mammary carcinoma. Cancer 51:654–661.

Lloyd RV, Shapiro B, Sisson JS, Kalff V, Thompson NW, Beierwalter A (1984): An immunohistochemical study of pheochromocytomas. Arch Pathol Lab Med 108:541–544.

Lokich JJ, Ellenberg S, Gerson B (1984): Criteria for monitoring carcinoembryonic antigen: Variability of sequential assays at elevated levels. J Clin Oncol 2:181–186.

Long JC, Aisenberg AC, Zamecnik PC (1977): Chromatographic and electrophoretic analysis of an antigen in Hodgkin's disease tissue cultures. J Natl Cancer Inst 58:223–227.

Loose JH, Damjanov I, Harris H (1984): Identity of the neoplastic alkaline phosphatase as revealed with monoclonal antibodies to the placental form of the enzyme. Am J Clin Pathol 82:137–177.

Lopez DM, Parks WP, Silverman MA, Distasio JA (1981): Lymphoproliferative responses to mouse mammary tumor virus in lymphocyte subsets of breast cancer patients. J Natl Cancer Inst 67:353–358.

Luger TA, Linkesch W, Knobler R, Konoschka EM (1983): Serial determination of serum ferritin levels in patients with malignant melanoma. Oncology 40:263–267.

Luk GD, Baylin SB (1984): Ornithine decarboxylase as a biologic marker in familial colonic polyposis. N Engl J Med 311:80–83.

Lüning B, Wiklund B, Redelius P, Björklund B (1980): Biochemical properties of tissue polypeptide antigen. Biochim Biophys Acta 624:90–101.

Luster W, Gropp C, Sostmann H, Kalbfleisch H, Havemann K (1982): Demonstration of immunoreactive calcitonin in sera and tissues of lung cancer patients. Eur J Cancer Clin Oncol 18:1275–1283.

Lüthgens M, Schlegel G (1981): Verlaufskontrolle mit Tissue Polypeptide Antigen und Carcinoembryonalem Antigen in der radioonkologischen Nachsorge und Therapie. Tumor Diagnostik 2:179–188.

Lüthgens M, Schlegel G (1983): Combined use of carcinoembryonic antigen and tissue polypeptide antigen in oncologic therapy and surveillance. In Nieburgs HE, Birkmayer GD, Klavins JV (eds): "Human Tumor Markers: Biological Basis and Clinical Relevance." New York: Alan R. Liss, pp 51–59.

Ma J, DeBoer WG, Ward HA, Nairn RC (1980): Another oncofetal antigen in colonic carcinoma. Br J Cancer 41:325–328.

Mackie RM, Campbell I, Turbitt ML (1984): Use of NK1C3 monoclonal antibody in the assessment of benign and malignant melanocytic lesions. J Clin Pathol 37:367–372.

Macleod RM, Whybrew WD, Bucovaz ET (1984) Cancer detection: Investigation of the role of B-protein in malignancies. Fed. Proc. 43:1751.

Madedden G, Langer M, Dettori G, Costanza C (1980): Role of serum carcinoembryonic antigen in preoperative diagnosis of cancer in patients with thyroid nodules. Cancer 45:2607–2610.

Maeyama M, Tayama C, Inoue S, Tajima C, Onizuka Y, Tanaka N, Nakayama M, Iwamasa T (1984): Serial serum determination on alpha-fetoprotein as a marker of the effect of postoperative chemotherapy in ovarian endodermal sinus tumor. Gynecol Oncol 17: 104–116.

Magnani JL, Nilsson B, Brockhaus M, Zopf D, Steplewski Z, Koprowski H, Ginsburg V (1982): A monoclonal antibody-defined antigen associated with gastrointestinal cancer in a ganglioside containing sialylated lacto-N-fucopentose II. J Biol Chem 257:14365–14369.

Mahaley MS Jr (1971): Immunological studies with human gliomas. J Neurosurg 24: 458–459.

Maidment BW, Papsidero LD, Nemoto T, Chu TM (1981): Recovery of immunologically reactive antibodies and antigens from breast cancer immune complexes by preparative isoelectric focusing. Cancer Res 41:795–800.

Malcolm AJ, Shipman RC, and Levy JG (1982): Detection of a tumor-associated antigen on the surface of human myelogenous leukemia cells. J Immunol 129:2599–2603.

Mambo NC (1983): Isoantigen states in condyloma acuminata of the uterine cervix. An immunoperoxidase study. Am J Clin Pathol 79:178–181.

Manes C (1974): Phasing of gene products during development. Cancer Res 34:2044–2052.

Mann DL, Halterman R, Leventhal B (1974): Acute leukemia-associated antigens. Cancer 34:1446–1451.

Mantovani G, Manca MA, Cossu F, Proto E, Taglieri G, Mirigliani F, Gaspardini G (1981): Evaluation of the specificity of the leukocyte migration inhibition test against histologically homologous and heterologous neoplastic antigens in cancer patients. Tumori 67:169–175.

Maruyama H, Mori T, Inaji H, Chu TM, Kosaki G (1983): Differential distribution of the pancreatic cancer-associated antigen (PCAA) and pancreatic tissue antigen (PaA) in pancreatic and gastrointestinal cancer tissues. Ann NY Acad Sci 417:240–250.

Matsumoto Y, Suzuki T, Asada I, Ozawa K, Tobe T, Hojno I (1982): Clinical classification of hepatoma in Japan according to serial changes in serum alpha-fetoprotein levels. Cancer 49:354–360.

Matthews JB, Mason GI (1983): Granular cell myoblastoma: An immunoperoxidase study using a variety of antisera to human carcinoembryonic antigen. Histopathology 7:77–82.

Mazoujian G, Pinkus GS, Haagensen DE Jr (1984): Extramammary Paget's disease—Evidence for an apocrine origin. An immunoperoxidase study of gross cystic disease fluid protein-15, carcinoembryonic antigen, and keratin proteins. Am J Surg Pathol 8:42–50.

McCabe RP, Haspel MV, Hoover HC, Pomato N, Peters L, Hanna MG Jr (1984): Human monoclonal antibodies in colorectal cancer. Fed Proc 43:1512.

McCluskey DR (1982): Fetal and oncofetal antigens—Regulators of immune reactions. Med Hypoth 8:627–634.

McCoy JL, Jerome LF, Dean JH, Perlin E, Oldham RK, Char DH, Cohen MH, Felix EL, Herberman RB (1975): Inhibition of leukocyte migration by tumor-associated antigens in soluble extracts of human malignant melanoma. J Natl Cancer Inst 55:19–24.

McCoy JL, Jerome LF, Anderson C, Cannon GB, Alford TC, Connor RJ, Oldham RK, Herberman RB (1976): Leukocyte migration inhibition by soluble extracts of MCF-7 tissue culture cell line derived from breast carcinoma. J Natl Cancer Inst 57:1045–1049.

McFarlane IG, Bullock S, Melia W, Williams R (1980): Hepatocellular oncofetal antigen: Relationship to normal human fetal ferritin. Gut 21:A899.

McGee JO, Woods JC, Ashall F, Branwell ME, Harris H (1982): A new marker for human cancer cells. 2. Immunohistochemical detection of the Ca antigen in human tissue with the Ca 1 antibody. Lancet 2:7–10.

McIntire KR, Waldmann TA, Moertel CG, Go VLW (1975): Serum α-fetoprotein in patients with neoplasms of gastrointestinal tract. Cancer Res 35:991–996.

Melia WM, Bullock S, Johnson PJ, Williams R (1983): Serum ferritin in hepatocellular carcinoma. A comparison with alpha fetoprotein. Cancer 51:2112–2115.

Mendelsohn G, Gessell M, Berger CL, Baylin SB (1984): Relationship of carcinoembryonic antigen and calcitonin immunoreactivity to tumor virulence in medullary thyroid carcinoma. Lab Invest 50:39A.

Mesa-Tejada R, Fierer JA, Klavins JV, Weiss M, Berkman JI (1972a): Presence of fetal antigens in human malignant neoplasms as demonstrated by immunofluorescence microscopy. In Anderson NG, Coggin JH Jr, Cole E, Holliman JW (eds): "Embryonic and Fetal Antigens in Cancer." Springfield, VA: National Technical Information Service, U.S. Department of Commerce, Conf.-720208, pp 177–180.

Mesa-Tejada R, Weiss M, Klavins JV, and Berkman JI (1972b): Human carcinoma antigens cross reacting with antiplacental antibodies. Fed Proc 31:639.

Mesa-Tejada R, Bhattacharyya J, Rorat E, Fenoglio CM, Klavins JV (1977): A widely cross-reacting tumor associated antigen in carcinoma of pancreas. Fed Proc 36:1075.

Mesa-Tejada R, Keydar I, Ramanarayanan M, Ohno T, Fenoglio C, Spiegelman S (1978): Detection in human breast carcinoma of an antigen immunologically related to a group-specific antigen of mouse mammary tumor virus. Proc Natl Acad Sci USA 75:1529–1533.

Mesa-Tejada R, Oster MW, Fenoglio CM, Magidson J, Spiegelman S (1982): Diagnosis of primary breast carcinoma through immunohistochemical detection of antigen related to mouse mammary tumor virus in metastatic lesions: A report of two cases. Cancer 49: 261–268.

Messing EM, Bubbers JE, Whitmore KE, de Kernion JB, Nestor MS, Fahey JL (1984): Murin hybridoma antibodies against human transitional carcinoma-associated antigens. J Urol 132:167–172.

Metzgar RS, Mohanakumar T (1977): Serologic studies of the diagnosis and nosology of human leukemia. Am J Clin Pathol 68:699–705.

Metzgar RS, Mohanakumar T, Bolognesi DP (1976): Relationship between membrane antigens of human leukemic cells and oncogenic RNA virus structural components. J Exp Med 143:47–63.

Michelson JB, Felberg NT, Shields JA (1976): Fetal antigens in retinoblastoma. Cancer 37:719–723.

Micksche M, Kokron O, Wolf A (1982): Radioimmunoassay (RIA) for a human lung cancer marker. Cancer Det Prev 5:256.

Midiri G, Amanti C, Consorti F, Benedetti M, Del Buono S, Di Tonto U, Castagna G, Peronace L, Di Paola M (1983): Usefulness of preoperative CEA levels in the assessment of colorectal cancer patient stage. J Surg Oncol 22:257–260.

Miettinen M, Holthofer H, Lehto VP, Miettinen A, Virtanen I (1983): Ulex europaeus I lectin as a marker for tumors derived from endothelial cells. Am J Clin Pathol 79:32–36.

Mihalev A, Tzingilev D, Sirakov LM (1976): Radioimmunoassay of alpha-fetoprotein in the serum of patients with leukemia and malignant melanoma. Neoplasma 23:103–107.

Millán JL, Stigbrand T (1983): Antigenic determinants of human placental and testicular placental-like alkaline phosphatases as mapped by monoclonal antibodies. Eur J Biochem 136:1–7.

Miller AL, Tom BH (1980): Human colon tumor-associated antigens detected with a monoclonal antibody. Proc Am Assoc Cancer Res 21:221.

Minei M, Yamana Y, Ohnishi Y (1983): Carcinoembryonic antigen and alpha fetoprotein levels in retinoblastoma. Jpn J Opthalmol 27:185–192.

Minowada J, Janossy G, Greaves MF, Tsubota T, Srivastava BI, Morikawa S, Tatsumi E (1978): Expression of an antigen associated with acute lymphoblastic leukemia in human leukemia-lymphoma cell lines. J Natl Cancer Inst 60:1269–1277.

Minton JP (1982): Colon cancer: Special surgical considerations. Cancer 50:2624–2626.

Mitchell KF, Fuhrer JP, Steplewski Z, Koprowski H (1981): Structural characterization of the "melanoma specific" antigen detected by monoclonal antibody 691I5NU-4-B. Mol Immunol 18:207–218.

Mitomi T, Nakasaki H, Tajima T, Ogoshi K, Tsuda M, Katsunuma T (1982): The role of a serum DNA-binding protein (64DP) in the diagnosis of malignant neoplasms. Int Adv Surg Oncol 5:245–259.

Miyauchi T, Yonezawa S, Takamura T, Chiba T, Tejima S, Ozawa M, Sato E, Muramatsu T (1982): A new fucosyl antigen expressed on colon adenocarcinoma cells. Nature 299:168–169.

Mohanakumar T, Giedin MA, Baker MA, Roncari DA, Taub RN (1981): Human acute myelogenous leukemia-associated antigens defined by a monkey antiserum to glycoproteins shed from leukemia myeloblasts. Leuk Res 5:11–17.

Mohanakumar T, Coffey TW, Vaughn MP, Russell EC, Conrad D (1983): Characterization of non-human primate antisera to acute lymphoblastic leukemia (ALL): Evidence for unique antigen(s) on childhood ALL of "T" phenotype. Blood 61:66–70.

Mohr JA, Nordquist RE, Rhoades ER, Coalson RE, Coalson JJ (1974): Alveolar cell carcinoma-like antigen and antibodies in patients with alveolar cell carcinoma and other cancers. Cancer Res 34:1904–1007.

Mohr JA, Nordquist RE, Coalson RE, Rhoades ER, Coalson JJ (1975): Lymphocyte-associated antigens in patients with alveolar cell carcinoma. J Lab Clin Med 86:490–493.

Monteiro JC, Ferguson KM, McKinna JA, Greening WP, Neville AM (1984): Ectopic production of human chorionic gonadotropin-like material by breast cancer. Cancer 53: 957–962.

Moody TW, Pert CB, Gazdar AF, Carney DN, Minna JD (1981): High levels of intracellular bombesin characterize human small-cell lung carcinoma. Science 214:1246–1248.

Moore M, Witherow PJ, Price CHG, Clough SA (1973): Detection by immunofluorescence of intracytoplasmic antigens in cell lines derived from human sarcomas. Int J Cancer 12:428–437.

Moore MR, Garrett PR Jr, Walton KN, Waldmann TA, McIntire RK, Counts P, Vogel CL (1978): Evaluation of human chorionic gonadotropin and alpha fetoprotein in benign and malignant testicular disorders. Surg Gynecol Obstet 147:167–174.

Mordasini C, Riesen W, Morell A (1982): Serum beta 2-microglobulin and other tumor associated antigens in patients with bronchogenic carcinoma. Lung 160:187–194.

Morgan AC, Reisfeld RA (1982): Detection and characterization of a monoclonal antibody-defined melanoma associated antigen with circulating immune complexes in normal donor sera. Fed Proc 41:410.

Morgan AC, Galloway DR, Jensen FC, Giovanella BC, Reisfeld RA (1981): Immunohistochemical delineation of an oncofetal antigen on normal and simian virus 40-transformed human fetal melanocytes. Proc Natl Acad Sci USA 78:3834–3838.

Morgan AC Jr, Crane MM, Rossen RD (1984): Measurement of a monoclonal antibody-defined melanoma associated antigen in human sera: Correlation of circulating antigen levels with tumor burden. J Natl Cancer Inst 72:243–249.

Mori W, Asakawa H, Taguchi T (1975): Antiserum against leukemia cell ferritin as a diagnostic tool for malignant neoplasms. J Natl Cancer Inst 55:513–518.

Morizane T, Kumagai N, Tsuchimoto K, Watanabe T, Tsuchiya M (1980): Specific immunodiagnosis of hepatoma by tube leukocyte adherence inhibition assay and a modified method of repeated tube leukocyte adherence inhibition assay. Cancer Res 40:2928–2934.

Moroz C, Kan M, Chaimof C, Marcus H, Kupfer B, Cuckles HS (1984): Ferritin-bearing lymphocytes in the diagnosis of breast cancer. Cancer 54:84–89.

Morton DL, Malmgren RA (1968): Human osteosarcomas: Immunologic evidence suggesting an associated infectious agent. Science 162:1279–1281.

Morton DL, Malmgren RA, Holmes EC, Ketcham AS (1968): Demonstration of antibodies against human malignant melanoma by immunofluorescence. Surgery 64:233–240.

Morton LC, Taub R, Diamond A, Lane M, Cooper G, Leder P (1984): Mapping of the human Blym-1 transforming gene activated in Burkitt lymphomas to chromosome 1. Science 223:173–175.

Mounts P, Shah KV, Kashima H (1982): Viral etiology of juvenile- and adult-onset squamous papilloma of the larynx. Proc Natl Acad Sci USA 79:5425–5429.

Mufti GJ, Hamblin TJ, Stevens J (1982): Basic isoferritin and hypercalcemia in renal cell carcinoma. J Clin Pathol 35:1008–1010.

Mughal AW, Hortobagyi GN, Fritsche HA, Buzdar AU, Yap H-Y, Blumenschein GR (1983): Serial plasma carcinoembryonic antigen measurements during treatment of metastatic breast cancer. JAMA 249:1881–1886.

Mukai M, Iri H, Torikata, C, Kageyama K, Morikawa Y, Shimizu K (1984): Immunoperoxidase demonstration of a new muscle protein (z-protein) in myogenic tumors as a diagnostic aid. Am J Pathol 114:164–170

Mukherji B, Hirshaut Y (1973): Evidence for fetal antigen in human sarcoma. Science 181:440–442.

Mulder H, Hackeng WH, Silberbusch J, Den Ottolander GJ, Van der Meer C (1981): Value of serum calcitonin estimation in clinical oncology. Br J Cancer 43:786–792.

Mulshine JL, Cuttitta F, Bibro M, Fedorko J, Fargion S, Little C, Carney DN, Gazdar AF, Minna JD (1983): Monoclonal antibodies that distinguish non-small cell from small cell lung cancer. J Immunol 131:497–502.

Munjal D, Rosano J, McFadden J, Picken J, Pritchard J (1983): Combined measurement of lipid-bound sialic acid (LSA) and carcinoembryonic antigen (CEA) in cancer patients. Fed Proc 42:403.

Munjal DD, Ugen KE, Hill JR (1981): Concurrent measurement of UDP-galactosyltransferase and carcinoembryonic antigen levels in cancer patients. Fed Proc 40:832.

Munther AS, Ramey WG, Hasim GA, Fitzpatrick HF (1980): Antigenic cross-recognition by T-lymphocytes from patients with cystosarcoma phyllodes and adenocarcinoma of the breast. Proc Am Assoc Cancer Res 21:243.

Muto Y, Omori M (1981): A novel cellular retinoid-binding protein, F-type, in hepatocellular carcinoma. Ann NY Acad Sci 359:91–103.

Nadji M, Morales AR, Ziegles-Weissman J, Penneys NS (1981a): Keposi's sarcoma: Immunohistologic evidence for an endothelial origin. Arch Pathol Lab Med 105:274–275.

Nadji M, Tabei SZ, Castro A, Chu TM, Murphy GP, Wang MC, Morales AR (1981b): Prostatic-specific antigens: An immunohistologic marker for prostatic neoplasms. Cancer 48:1229–1232.

Nadji M, Ganjei P, Shimano T, Chu TM, Morales AR (1982): Pancreatic carcinoma associated antigen: A marker for pancreatic carcinoma. Lab Invest 46:60A.

Nadkarin JS, Nadkarin JJ, Gollerkeri MP (1973): Search for tumor specific reactivity in human leukemias. Indian J Cancer 10:338–345.

Nadler LM, Stashenko P, Hardy R, Schlossman SF (1980): A monoclonal antibody defining a lymphoma-associated antigen in man. J Immunol 125:570–577.

Naito K, Yamaguchi H, Horibe K, Shiku H, Takahashi T, Suzuki S, Yamada K (1983): Autologous and allogeneic typing of human leukemia cells: Definition of surface antigens restricted to lymphocytic leukemia cells. Proc Natl Acad Sci US 80:2341–2345.

Nakai M (1983): Electron microscopic observation of ATLV (Adult T-Cell Leukemia Associated Virus). Gan To Kagaku Ryoho 10:663–668.

Nakajima T, Watanabe S, Sato Y, Kameya T, Shimosato Y (1981): Immunohistochemical demonstration of S 100 protein in human malignant melanoma and pigmented nevi. Gan 72:335–336.

Nakajima T, Watanabe S, Sato Y, Kameya T, Hirota T, Shimosata Y (1982): An immunoperoxidase study of S-100 protein distribution in normal and neoplastic tissues. Am J Surg Pathol 6:715–727.

Nakanishi I, Kawahara E, Kajikawa K, Miwa A, Terahata S (1982): Hyaline globules in yolk sac tumor. Histochemical, immunohistochemical and electron microscopic studies. Acta Pathol Jpn 32:733–739.

Nakano H, Yamamoto F, Neville C, Evans D, Mizuno T, Perucho M (1984): Isolation of transforming sequences of two human lung carcinomas: Structural and functional analysis of the activated c-K-ras oncogenes. Proc Natl Acad Sci USA 81:71–75.

Nakatsu H, Kobayashi I, Onishi Y, Igawa M, Ito H, Tahara E, Nihira H (1984): ABO (H) blood group antigens and carcinoembryonic antigens as indicators of malignant potential in patients with transitional cell carcinoma of the bladder. J Urol 131:252–257.

Nakazato Y, Ishizeki J, Takahashi K, Yamaguchi H, Kamei T, Mori T (1982): Localization of S-100 protein and glial fibrillary acidic protein-related antigen in pleomorphic adenoma of the salivary glands. Lab Invest 46:621–626.

Nap M, Keuning H, Burtin P, Oosterhuis JW, Fleuren G (1984): CEA and NCA in benign and malignant breast tumors. Am J Clin Pathol 82:526–534.

Natali PG, Imai K, Wilson BS, Bigoti A, Cavaliere R, Pellegrino MA, Ferrone S (1981): Structural properties and tissue distribution of the antigen recognized by the monoclonal antibody 653.40 S to human melanoma cells. J Natl Cancer Inst 67:591–601.

Nathrath WBJ, Heidenkummer P (1983): Lokalisation von "Tissue Polypeptide Antigen" (TPA) in normalen und neoplastischen Geweben des Menschen. Verh Dtsch Ges Pathol 67:701.

Nathrath WBJ, Arnholdt H, Wilson PD (1982): Keratin luminal epithelial antigen and carcinoembryonic antigen in human urinary bladder carcinomas. Pathol Res Pract 175: 279–288.

Neel HB, Pearson GR, Weiland LH, Taylor WF, Goepfert HH, Pilch BZ, Goodman M, Lanier AP, Huang AT, Hyams VJ, Levine PH, Henle G, Henle W (1983): Application of Epstein-Barr virus serology to the diagnosis and staging of North American patients with nasopharyngeal carcinoma. Otolaryngol Head Neck Surg 91:255–262.

Negishi Y, Mutai Y, Akiya K, Fujiwara Y, Singh G (1984): Tumor associated antigen in ovarian carcinoma. Nippon Sanka Fujinka Gakkai Zasshi 36:126–132.

Newlands ES, Begent RH, Rustin GJ, Parker D, Bagshaw KD (1983): Further advances in the management of malignant teratomas of the testis and other sites. Lancet 1:948–951.

Nilsson B, Wahren B, Esposti PL, Edsmyr F (1982): Prediction of survival and recurrence in bladder carcinoma. Urol Res 10:109–113.

Nishimura S, Shindo-Okada N, Kasai H, Kuchino Y, Noguchi S, Iigo M, Hoshi A (1982): Characterization and analysis of oncofetal tRNA and its possible application for cancer diagnosis and therapy. Recent Results Cancer Res 84:401–412.

Nitti D, Farini R, Grassi F, Di Mario F, Piccoli A, Vianello F, Farinati F, Favretti F, Lise M, Naccarato R (1983): Carcinoembryonic antigen in gastric juice collected during endoscopy. Value in detecting high-risk patients and gastric cancer. Cancer 52:2334–2337.

Norton JA, Doppman JL, Brennan MF (1980): Localization and resection of clinically inapparent medullary carcinoma of the thyroid. Surgery 87:616–622.

Nudelman E, Hakomori S, Kannagi R, Levery S, Yeh MY, Hellström KE, Hellström I (1982): Characterization of a human melanoma-associated ganglioside antigen defined by a monoclonal antibody, 4.2. J Biol Chem 257:12752–12756.

Nudelman E, Kannagi R, Hakomori S, Parsons M, Lipinski M, Wiels J, Fellous M, Tursz T (1983): A glycolipid antigen associated with Burkitt lymphoma defined by a monoclonal antibody. Science 220:509–511.

O'Brien P, Gozzo JJ, Monaco AP (1980): Detection of a 50,000 dalton tumor associated antigen(s) in urine from patients with bladder cancer. Fed Proc 39:351.

Ochi H, Kim U, Holyoke ED, Sandberg AA (1983): Cytogenetic analysis of primary large bowel cancers. Proc Am Assoc Cancer Res 24:495.

Odell WD, Wolfsen AR, Bachelot I, Hirose FM (1979): Ectopic production of lipotropin by cancer. Am J Med 66:631–638.

Oehr P, Derigs G, Altmann R (1981): Evaluation and characterization of tumor-associated antigens by conversion of inverse distribution function values into specificity-sensitivity diagrams. Tumor Diagn 2:283–290.

Ogier C, Giannoulis N, Jacobs A, Reizenstein PG (1984): The use of serum ferritin to identify good and bad prognosis groups in acute myeloid leukemia. Hematologica 69:111–112.

Oguchi H, Homma T, Kawa S, Nagata A, Furuta S, Fukui H (1984): A pancreatic oncofetal antigen (POA): Its characterization and application for enzyme immunoassay. Cancer Det Prev 7:51–58.

Oji M, Furue M, Tamaki K (1984): Serum carcinoembryonic antigen level in Paget's disease. Br J Dermatol 110:211–213.

Okagaki T, Clark BA, Zachow KR, Twiggs LB, Ostrow RS, Pass F, Faras AJ (1984): Presence of human papillomavirus in verrucous carcinoma (Ackerman) of the vagina. Arch Pathol Lab Med 108:567–570.

Okano T, Kawaoi A, Nemoto N, Ishibashi H, Sato H, Shikata T, Hirata Y (1982): Is epidermal growth factor (EGF) the tumor marker of various human malignancies? J Histochem Cytochem 30:556.

Olsson L, Andreasen RB, Ost A, Christensen B, Biberfeld P (1984): Antibody producing human-human hybridomas. II. Derivation and characterization of an antibody specific for human leukemia cells. J Exp Med 159:537–550.

Ona FV, Zamcheck N, Dhar P, Moore T, Kupchick HZ (1973): Carcinoembryonic antigen (CEA) in the diagnosis of pancreatic cancer. Cancer 31:324–327.

O'Neill G, Gold P, Murgita RA (1981): Immunoregulatory effect of human alpha-fetoprotein on T-lymphocyte activation induced by autologous cells. Fed Proc 40:1077.

Order SE, Colgan J, Hellman S (1974): Distribution of fast- and slow-migrating Hodgkin's tumor-associated antigens. Cancer Res 34:1182–1186.

Ordonez NG, Manning JT Jr, Hanssen G (1983): Alpha-1-antitrypsin in islet cell tumors of the pancreas. Amer J Clin Pathol 80:277–282.

Ossowski L, Vassalli J-D (1978): Plasminogen activator in normal and malignant cells: A comparison of enzyme levels and of hormonal responses. In Ruddon RW (ed): "Biological Markers of Neoplasia: Basic and Applied Aspects." New York: Elsevier/North-Holland, pp 473–478.

Ozaki HS, Yoneyama T, Kodama T, Hoshino K (1982): Correlation between nuclear DNA model patterns and preoperative plasma carcinoembryonic antigen levels in lung cancer patients. Jpn J Clin Oncol 12:99–107.

Pagé M, Dalifard E, Drouin R, Bertrand G, Daver A, Esperandieu O (1984): Immunohistological studies of human sarcomas with monoclonal antibodies. Fed Proc 43:1510.

Paiva J, Damjanov I, Lange PH, Harris H (1983): Immunohistochemical localization of placental-like alkaline phosphatase in testis and germ-cell tumors using mononclonal antibodies. Am J Pathol 111:156–165.

Pak KY, Blaszczyk M, Steplewski Z, Koprowski H (1983): Identification and isolation of a common tumor-associated molecule using monoclonal antibody. Mol Immunol 20: 1369–1377.

Palazzo S, Liguori V, Molinari B, Greco LM, Mancini V (1984): The role of carcinoembryonic antigen in the postmastectomy follow-up of primary breast cancer and in the prognostic evaluation of disseminated breast cancer. Tumori 70:57–59.

Palker TJ, Scearce RM, Miller SE, Popovic M, Bolognesi DP, Gallo RC, Haynes BF (1984): Monoclonal antibodies against human T cell leukemia-lymphoma virus (HTLV) p24 internal core protein. Use as diagnostic probes and cellular localization of HTLV. J Exp Med 159:1117–1131.

Pandolfi F, Luzi G, Tozzi MC, Aiuti F (1977): Preparation, purification and in vitro properties of a serum against human lymphoblastic leukemia-associated antigens. Acta Haematol 57:257–265.

Pant KD, Dahlman HL, Goldenberg DM (1977): A putatively new antigen (CSAp) associated with gastrointestinal and ovarian neoplasia. Immunol Commun 6:411–422.

Pant KD, Shochat D, Nelson MD, Goldenberg DM (1982): Colon-specific antigen-p(CSAp). I: Initial clinical evaluation as a marker for colorectal cancer. Cancer 50:919–926.

Papenhausen PR, Emeson EE, Croft CB, Borowiecki B (1984): Ferritin-bearing lymphocytes in patients with cancer. Cancer 53:267–271.

Parada LF, Tabin CJ, Shih C, Weinberg RA (1982): Human EJ bladder carcinoma oncogene is homologue of Harvey sarcoma virus ras gene. Nature 297:474–479.

Paradinas FJ, Melia WM, Wilkinson ML, Portmann B, Johnson PJ, Murray-Lyon IM, Williams R (1982): High serum vitamin B_{12} binding capacity as a marker of the fibrolamellar variant of hepatocellular carcinoma. Br Med J 285:840–842.

Parsa I, Sutton A, Chen CK, Delbridge C (1982): Monoclonal antibody for identification of human duct cell carcinoma of pancreas. Cancer Lett 17:217–222.

Parsons RG, Hoch JA (1976): Purification and identification of a human-serum DNA-binding protein associated with malignant diseases. Eur J Biochem 71:1–8.

Parsons RG, Kowal R (1978): Detection of a new malignancy-associated DNA-binding protein in human serum. Proc Am Assoc Cancer Res 19:99.

Parsons RG, Hoch JA, Longmire RL, Kowal R (1978): Serum DNA-binding proteins. In Ruddon RW (ed): "Biological Markers of Neoplasia: Basic and Applied Aspects." New York: Elsevier, pp. 385–396.

Parsons RG, Todd HD, Kowal R (1979): Isolation and identification of a human serum fibronectin-like protein elevated during malignant disease. Cancer Res. 39:4341–4345.

Pasternak G, Schlott B, Reinhofer J, Gryschek G, von Broen B, Albrecht S (1982): Reactivity in neoplasia, preneoplasia, and frequency of lymphocytes against fetal extracts: Cross-reactions between man and mouse. J Natl Cancer Inst 69:997–1004.

Pattengale PK, Taylor CR, Chir B, Engvall E, Ruoslahti E (1980): Direct tissue visualization of normal cross-reacting antigen in neoplastic granulocytes. Am J Clin Pathol 73:351–355.

Payne JE, Dent O, Chapuis PH, Meyer HJ, Sutherland MA, Ruwoldt A (1983): Leukocyte adherence inhibition and carcinoembryonic antigen in combination for diagnosis of colorectal cancer. J Surg Oncol 22:212–215.

Pelicci P-G, Lanfrancone L, Brathwaite MD, Wolman SR, Dalla-Favera R (1984): Amplification of the c-myb oncogene in a case of human acute myelogenous leukemia. Science 224:117–121.

Penneys NS, Nadji M, Ziegels-Weismann J, Ketabchi M, Morales AR (1982): Carcinoembryonic antigen in sweat-gland carcinoma. Cancer 50:1608–1611.

Perras J, Cramer J, Bishop R, Averette H, Sevin BU (1983): Detection of increased levels of cysteinyl proteinase activity in urine of gynecological cancer patients. Proc Am Assoc Cancer Res 23:513.

Persijn JP (1982): Carcino-embryonic antigen (CEA) during treatment of recurrent or inoperable tumours of the digestive tract. Neth J Med 25:360–364.

Pesando JM, Ritz J, Levine H, Terhorst C, Lazarus H, Schlossman SF (1980): Human leukemia-associated antigen: Relation to a family of surface glycoproteins. J Immunol 124:2794–2799.

Pflüger KH, Gropp C, Havemann K (1982): Ectopically produced calcitonin in human neuroblastoses. Klin Wochenscher 60:667–672.

Pfreundschuh M, Shiker H, Takahashi T, Ueda R, Ransohoff J, Oettgen HF, Old LJ (1978): Serological analysis of cell surface antigens of malignant human brain tumors. Proc Natl Acad Sci USA 75:5122–5126.

Pilch YH, Fritze D, Kern DH (1976): Mediation of immune responses to human tumor antigens with "immune" RNA. In Wybran J, Staquet MJ (eds): "Clinical Tumor Immunology" New York: Pergamon Press, pp 169–190.

Pimentel E (1983): Hormones as tumor markers. In Nieburgs HE, Birkmayer GD, Klavins JV (eds): "Human Tumor Markers: Biological Basis and Clinical Relevance." New York: Alan R. Liss, pp 87–93.

Plowman GD, Brown JP, Enns CA, Schroder J, Nikinmaa B, Sursman HH, Hellström KE, Hellström I (1983): Assignment of the gene for human melanoma-associated antigen P97 to chromosome 3. Nature 303:70–72.

Podolsky DK, McPhee MS, Alpert E, Warshaw AL, Isselbacher KJ (1981): Galactosyltransferase isoenzyme II in the detection of pancreatic cancer: Comparison with radiologic, endoscopic and serologic tests. N Engl J Med 304:1313–1318.

Pohl AL, Francesconi M, Ganzinger UC, Graninger W, Lenzhofer RS, Moser KV (1983): Present value of tumor markers in the clinic. In Nieburgs HE, Birkmayer GD, Klavins JV (eds): "Human Tumor Markers: Biological Basis and Clinical Relevance." New York: Alan R. Liss, pp 7–20.

Pollack MS, Slimp GH, Sokal JE (1977): The serological detection of leukemia-associated antigens in chronic leukemia: Correlation with disease status. Am J Hematol 3:93–104.

Pontes JE, Chu TM, Slack N, Karr J, Murphy GP (1982): Serum prostatic antigen measurement in localized prostatic cancer: Correlation with clinical course. J Urol 128:1216–1218.

Posner LE, Robert-Guroff M, Kalyanaraman WS, Poiesz BJ, Ruscetti FW, Fossieck B, Bunn PA, Minna JD, Gallo RC (1981): Natural antibodies to the human T cell lymphoma virus in patients with cutaneous T cell lymphoma. J Exp Med 154:333–346.

Posnett, DN, Chiorazzi, N, Kunkel HG (1982): Monoclonal antibodies with specificity for hairy cell leukemia cells. J Clin Invest. 70:254–261.

Posnett DN, Marboe CC, Knowles DM, Jaffe EA, Kunkel HG (1984): A membrane antigen (HCI) selectively present in hairy cell leukemia cells, endothelial cells, and epidermal basal cells. J Immunol 132:2700–2702.

Prat J, Bhan AK, Dickerrsin GR, Robboy SJ, Scully RE (1982): Hepatoid yolk sac tumor of the ovary (endodermal sinus tumor with hepatoid differentiation). A light microscopic ultrastructural and immunohistochemical study of seven cases. Cancer 50:2355–2368.

Prigogine T, Verbeet T, Schmerber J (1982): Carcinoembryonic antigen in pleural effusions: A diagnostic indicator. Eur J Respir Dis 63:141.

Priori ES, Wilbur JR, Dmochowski L (1971): Immunofluorescence tests on sera of patients with osteogenic sarcoma. J Natl Cancer Inst 46:1299–1308.

Pritchett TR, Skinner DG (1984): Embryonal carcinoma with falsely positive elevation of serum alpha-fetoprotein after curative therapy: A case report. J Urol 131:970–971.

Pullen S, Hersey P (1981): Reactivity of antisera to antigens of C-type viruses with leucocytes from patients with acute leukemia. Pathology 13:289–298.

Qian GX, Liu CK, Waxman S (1984): Abnormal isoelectric focusing patterns of serum galactosyltransferase activity in patients with liver neoplasia. Proc Soc Exp Biol Med 175:21–24.

Raghavan D, Sullivan AL, Peckham MJ, Neville AM (1982): Elevated serum alphafetoprotein and seminoma. Clinical evidence for a histologic continuum? Cancer 50:982–989.

Ramsey R, Lovins R, Hokama Y (1982): Histochemical localization of a new tumor-associated antigen. Fed Proc 41:555.

Raney B, Schlesinger H, Hummeler K (1978): Characterization of xenoantisera to human neuroblastoma (NBL) cells. Proc Am Assoc Cancer Res 19:182.

Rasmuson T, Bjork GR, Damber L, Holm SE, Jacobsson L, Jeppson A, Littbrand B, Stigbrand T, Westman G (1982): Evaluation of carcinoembryonic antigen, tissue polypeptide antigen, placental alkaline phosphatase, and modified nucleosides as markers in malignant lymphomas. Rec Results Cancer Res 84:331–343.

Reddi KK (1980): Clinical significance of human serum ribonuclease. In Kawai K (ed): "Early Diagnosis of Pancreatic Cancer." New York: Igaku-Shoin.

Redelius P, Lüning B, Björklund B (1980): Chemical studies of tissue polypeptide antigen (TPA). II. Partial amino acid sequences of cyanogen bromide fragments of TPA subunit B_1. Acta Chem Scand B 34:265–273.

Rees WV, Irie RF, Morton DL (1981): Oncofetal antigen-I: Distribution in human tumors. J Natl Cancer Inst 67:557–562.

Reilly CA Jr, Pritchard DJ, Biskis BO, Finkel MP (1972): Immunologic evidence suggesting a viral etiology of human osteosarcoma. Cancer 30:603–609.

Reitz MS, Poiesz BJ, Ruscetti FW, Gallo RC (1981a): Characterization and distribution of nucleic acid sequences of a novel type C retrovirus isolated from neoplastic human T lymphocytes. Proc Natl Acad Sci USA 78:1887–1891.

Reitz M, Wainberg M, Ruscetti F, Ceccherini-Nelli L, Gallo RC (1981b): HTLV, a type-C virus isolated from human T cell malignancies, is T-cell tropic. "RNA Viruses, May 20–24, 1981." Cold Spring Harbor, NY. Cold Spring Harbor Laboratory.

Renner IG, Chlebowski R, Bateman J, Douglas AP (1979): A comparison of carcinoembryonic antigen (CEA) and serum ribonuclease (S-RNase) in the diagnosis of malignant disease. Clin Res. 27:54.

Rickles FR, Edwards RL, Barb C, Cronlund M (1983): Abnormalitites of blood coagulation in patients with cancer. Fibrinopeptide A generation and tumor growth. Cancer 51:301–307.

Rinsho K, Aoyagi K (1982): Urinary hydroxyproline excretion as a marker of bone metastasis in prostatic cancer. Tohoku J Exp Med 137:461–462.

Ritts RE Jr, Del Villano BC, Go VL, Herberman RB, Klug TL, Zurawski VR Jr (1984): Initial clinical evaluation of an immunoradiometric assay for CA 19-9 using the NCI serum bank. Int J Cancer 33:339–345.

Robert-Guroff M, Nakao Y, Notake K, Ito Y, Sliski A, Gallo RC (1982): Natural antibodies to human retrovirus HTLV in a cluster of Japanese patients with adult T cell leukemia. Science 215:975–978.

Robertson AG, Read G (1982): The value of lactate dehydrogenase as a nonspecific tumour marker for seminoma of the testis. Br J Cancer 46:994–998.

Romano M, Cecco L, Cerra M, De Matteis A (1983): Polyamine excretion as prognostic marker in radiologic therapy of breast carcinoma in metastatic phase. Adv Polyamine Res 4:59–64.

Rosai J, Pinkus GS (1982): Immunohistochemical demonstration of epithelial differentiation in adamantinoma of the tibia. Am J Surg Pathol 6:427–434.

Rossiello R, Carriero MV, Giordano GG (1984): Distribution of ferritin, transferrin and lactoferrin in breast carcinoma tissue. J Clin Pathol 37:51–55.

Roti E, Robuschi G, Emanuele R, Bandini P, Russo A, Riva P, Galassi E, Guerra UP, Manfredi A, Bozzetti A, Guazzi AM, and Gnudi A (1982): The value of serum thyroglobulin measurement as a marker of cancer recurrence in the follow-up of patients previously treated for differentiated thyroid tumor. J Endocrinol Invest 5:43–46.

Rougier P, Calmettes C, Laplanche A, Travagli JP, Lefevre M, Parmentier C, Milhaud G, Tubiana M (1983): The values of calcitonin and carcinoembryonic antigen in the treatment and management of nonfamilial medullary thyroid carcinoma. Cancer 51:855–862.

Rozen A (1974): Neoplastic ovarian antigens: An investigative study. Ann Immunol 6:47–54.

Rozengur E, Collins M (1983): Molecular aspects of growth factor action: Receptors and intracellular signals. J Pathol 141:309–331.

Rubery ED, Doran JF, Thompson RJ (1982): Brain-type creatine kinase BB as a potential tumour marker—serum levels measured by radioimmunoassay in 1,015 patients with histologically confirmed malignancies. Eur J Cancer Clin Oncol 18:951–956.

Rudczynski AB, Dyer CA, Mortensen RF (1978): Detection of cell-mediated immune reactivity of breast cancer patients by the leukocyte adherence inhibition response to MCF-7 extracts. Cancer Res 38:3590–3594.

Rudman D, Chawla RK, Hendrickson LJ, Vogler WR, Sophianopoulos AJ (1976): Isolation of a novel glycoprotein (EDC1) from the urine of a patient with acute myelocytic leukemia. Cancer Res. 36:1837–1846.

Ruppert B, Maxwell B, Alpert E (1984): Monoclonal antibodies distinguishing ferritin from human pancreatic carcinoma and normal liver ferritin. Fed Proc 43:1420.

Rutherford JC, Walters BAJ, Cavaye G, Halliday WJ (1977): A modified leukocyte adherence inhibition test in the laboratory investigation of gastrointestinal cancer. Int J Cancer 19: 43–48.

Saad MF, Fritsche HA Jr, Samaan NA (1984): Diagnostic and prognostic values of carcinoembryonic antigen in medullary carcinoma of the thyroid. J Clin Endocrinol Metab 58:889–894.

Sadamori N, Nonaka H, Ichimaru M, Igarashi H, Hirota M, Sawada H (1981): Familial acute myelogenous leukemia associated with RNA virus and polymorphism of IQH+. Cancer Genet Cytogenet 4:23–30.

Sadananda B, Natarajan RS, Vittal C, Kalyankar GD (1980): Urinary polyamines in cancer. Indian J Cancer 17:220–225.

Said JW, Nash G, Lee M (1982): Immunoperoxidase localization of keratin proteins, carcinoembryonic antigen, and factor VIII in adenomatoid tumors: Evidence of a mesothelial derivation. Hum Pathol 13:1106–1108.

Said JW, Nash G, Banks-Schlegel S, Sassoon AF, Shintaku IP (1984): Localized fibrous mesothelioma. An immunohistochemical and electron microscopic study. Hum Pathol 15:440–443.

Saiki S, Kotake T, Kuroda M, Usami M, Kiyohara H, Miki T, Yoshida M, Matsumiya K, Kami O (1982): Carcinoma of the urachus: Report of two cases. Hinyokika Kiyo 28: 1271–1279.

Sakamoto J, Cordon-Cardo C, Friedman E, Finstad CL, Enker WE, Melamed MR, Shiku H, Lloyd KO, Oettgen HF, Old LF (1983): Antigens of normal and neoplastic human colonic mucosa cells (HCMC) defined by monoclonal antibodies (MAB). Proc Am Assoc Cancer Res 24:889.

Salinas FA, Wee KH, Silver HKB (1982): On the relationship of human oncofetal antigen (HOFA) to tumor burden in malignant melanoma (MM). Fed Proc. 41:553.

Salki S, Miki T, Hata T, Ogihara T, Shima K, Kumahara Y, Tsuchiyama M (1982): A case of pseudomyxoma peritonei with bilateral pleural metastases. Jpn J Clin Oncol 12:117–122.

Salvatore F, Colonna A, Costanzo F, Russo T, Esposito F, Climino F (1983a): Modified nucleosides in body fluids of tumor-bearing patients. Rec Res Cancer Res 84:360–377.

Salvatore F, Russo T, Colonna A, Cimino L, Mazzacca G, Cimino F (1983b): Pseudouridine determination in blood serum as tumor marker. Cancer Det Prev 6:531–536.

Sampson J, Wong L, Harris OD (1982): The role of Tennessee antigen in the diagnosis of gastrointestinal malignancy. Aust NZ J Surg 52:39–41.

Santos EP, Martin-Zanca D, Reddy EP, Pierotti MA, Della Porta G, Barbacid M (1984): Malignant activation of a K-ras oncogene in lung carcinoma but not in normal tissue of same patient. Science 223:661–664.

Saravis CA, Oh SK, Pusztaszeri G, Doos W, Zamcheck N (1978): Present status of zinc glycinate marker (ZGM). Cancer 42:1621–1625.

Sarin PS, Aoki T, Shibata A, Ohnishi Y, Aoyagi Y, Miyakoshi H, Emura I, Kalyanaraman VS, Robert-Guroff M, Popovic M, Sarngadharan M, Nowell PC, Gallo RC (1983): High incidence of human type-C retrovirus (HTLV) in family members of a HTLV-positive Japanese T-cell leukemia patient. Proc Natl Acad Sci USA 80:2370–2374.

Sato K, Raimondi AJ, Dray S, Molinaro GA (1978): Comparison of tumor-associated surface antigens on cells from medulloblastomas and from other neoplasms of the human nervous system. Childs Brain 4:83–84.

Satoh PS, Nelson SL, Hattler BG (1975): Fetal protein from human lung carcinoma: A heat stable fetal antigen which inhibits T cell rosette formation. Proc Am Assoc Cancer Res 16:59.

Sawabu N, Nakagen M, Ozaki K, Wakabayashi T, Toya D, Hattori N, Ishii M (1983): Clinical evaluation of specific gamma-GTP isoenzyme in patients with hepatocellular carcinoma. Cancer 51:327–331.

Scalabrino G, Ferioli ME (1982): Polyamines in mammalian tumors. Part II. Adv Cancer Res 36:1–102.

Schaffer R, Ormans W (1983): Immunohistochemical detection of factor VIII antigen in malignant hemangioendotheliomas of the thyroid. A contribution to histogenesis. Schweiz Med Wochenschr 113:601–605.

Schlom J, Wunderlich D, Teramoto YA (1980): Generation of human monoclonal antibodies reactive with human mammary carcinoma cells. Proc Natl Acad Sci USA 77:6841–6845.

Schneider J, Yamamoto N, Hinuma Y, Hunsmann G (1984): Sera from adult T-cell leukemia patients react with envelope and core polypeptides of adult T-cell leukemia virus. Virology 132:1–11.

Schwab U, Stein H, Gerdes H, Lemke H, Kirchner H, Schaadt M, Diehl V (1982): Production of a monoclonal antibody specific for Hodgkin and Sternberg-Reed cells of Hodgkin's disease and a subset of normal lymphoid cells. Nature 299:65–67.

Scully C (1982): Thymidine kinase acitivity in oral squamous cell carcinoma. J Oral Pathol 11:210–213.

Scurry J, de Boer WG (1983): Carcinoembryonic antigen in skin and related tumours as determined by immunohistological techniques. Pathology 15:379–384.

Sears HF, Koprowski H, Herlyn M, DelVillano B, Steplewski Z (1982): Serum antigen tumor marker for colon carcinoma. Hybridoma 1:217.

Seeger RC, Rosenblatt HM, Imai K, Ferrone S (1981): Common antigenic determinants on human melanoma, glioma, neuroblastoma, and sarcoma cells defined with monoclonal antibodies. Cancer Res 41:2714–2717.

Sega E, Mottolese M, Curcio CG, Citro G (1980): Specific blastogenesis response of peripheral blood lymphocytes from lung cancer patients to a fetal lung antigen. J Natl Cancer Inst 64:1001–1006.

Sehested M, Hou-Jensen K (1981): Factor VIII related antigen as an endothelial cell marker in benign and malignant diseases. Virchows Arch 391:217–225.

Seifert G, Caselitz J (1983): Tumor markers in parotid gland carcinomas: Immunohistochemical investigations. In Nieburgs, HE, Birkmayer GD, Klavins JV (eds): "Human Tumor Markers: Biological Basis and Clinical Relevance." New York: Alan R. Liss, pp 119–130.

Sen U, Guha S, Chawdhury JR (1983): Serum fucosyl transferase activity and serum fucose levels as diagnostic tools in malignancy. Acta Med Okayama 37:457–462.

Seon BK, Yoshizaki K, Negoro S, Minowada J, Pressman D (1980): Isolation of human thymus-leukemia associated antigens in a large scale. Fed Proc 39:351.

Seon BK, Negoro S, Barcos MP (1983): Monoclonal antibody that defines a unique human T-cell leukemia antigen. Proc Natl Acad Sci USA 80:845–849.

Sethi J, Hirshaut Y (1981): Characterization of human sarcoma antigen S. Br J Cancer 43: 261–266.

Shamberger P (1983): Evaluation of sialic acid levels as a tumor marker. Proc Am Assoc Cancer Res 23:491.

Sheikh KM, Lee YT, Quismorio FP, Friou GJ (1976): Antibodies to tumor associated antigens in breast carcinoma. Proc Am Assoc Cancer Res 17:150.

Sheikh KMA, Apuzzo MLJ, Kochsiek KR, Weiss MH (1977): Malignant glial neoplasms: Definition of a humoral host response to tumor-associated antigen(s). Yale J Biol Med 50:397–404.

Sheppard MN, Corrin B, Bennett MH, Marangos PJ, Bloom SR, Polak JM (1984): Immunocytochemical localization of neuron specific enolase in small cell carcinomas and carcinoid tumours of the lung. Histopathology 8:171–181.

Sherwin SA, Twardzik DR, Bohn WH, Cockley KD, Todaro GJ (1983): High-molecular-weight transforming growth factor activity in the urine of patients with disseminated cancer. Cancer Res 43:403–407.

Shi ZR, McIntyre LJ, Knowles BB, Soltzer D, Kim YS (1984): Expression of a carbohydrate differentiation antigen, stage-specific embryonic antigen 1, in human colonic adenocarcinoma. Cancer Res 44:1142–1147.

Shiku H, Takahashi T, Oettgen HF, Old LJ (1976): Cell surface antigens of human malignant melanoma: II. Serological typing with immune adherence assays and definition of two new surface antigens. J Exp Med 144:873–881.

Shillitoe EJ, Greenspan D, Greenspan JS, Silverman S Jr (1984): Antibody to early and late antigens of herpes simplex virus type 1 in patients with oral cancer. Cancer 54:266–273.

Shimano T, Loor RM, Papsidero LD, Kuriyama M, Vincent RG, Nemoto T, Holyoke ED, Barjian P, Douglass HO, Chu TM (1981): Isolation, characterization and clinical evaluation of a pancreas cancer-associated antigen. Cancer 47:1602–1613.

Shimano T, Mori T, Kitada M, Maruyama H, Kosaki G (1983): Purification and characterization of a pancreatic cancer-associated antigen (PCAA) from normal colonic mucosa. Ann NY Acad Sci 147:97–104.

Shimoyama M, Minato K, Tobinai K, Nagai M, Setoya T, Watanabe S, Hoshino H, Miwa M, Nagoshi H, Ichiki N, Fukushima N, Sugiura K, Funaki N (1983): Anti-ATLA (Antibody to adult T-cell leukemia-lymphoma virus-associated antigen)-negative adult T-cell leukemia-lymphoma. Jpn J Clin Oncol 13:245–256.

Shorthouse AJ, Carter SM, Ellison ML (1982): Tumour marker production in human bronchial carcinoma xenografts. Oncodev Biol Med 3:273–281.

Sikora K, Wright P (1981): Human monoclonal antibodies to lung-cancer antigens. Br J Cancer 43:696–700.

Silver HK, Murray RN, Worth AJ, Salinas FA, Spinelli JJ (1983): Prediction of malignant melanoma recurrence by serum N-acetylneuraminic acid. Int J Cancer 31:39–43.

Sindelar WF, Dresdale AR, Hadley NA (1983). Demonstration of tissue specific antigens shared by normal pancreas and pancreatic neoplasms. Experientia 39:87–89.

Singh B, Ragupathy R, Shaw ARE, Tews DG, Hamilton MS, Wegmann TG (1982): Characterization and cross-reactivity of human and mouse oncofetal antigens. Transplantation 33:156–162.

Skinner MS, Seckinger D (1979): Evaluation of beta subunit chorionic gonadotropin as an aid in diagnosis of trophoblastic disease. Ann Clin Lab Sci 9:347–352.

Smalley JR, Bystryn JC (1978): Purification of cell-surface glycoprotein from human melanoma. Fed Proc 37:1595.

Smith BJ, Wills MR, Savory J (1983): Prostaglandins and cancer. Ann Clin Lab Sci 13: 359–365.

Smith CJ, Ajdukiewicz A, Kelleher PC (1983): Concanavalin-A-affinity molecular heterogeneity of human hepatoma AFP and cord-serum AFP. Ann NY Acad Sci 417:69–74.

Smith HS, Riggs JL, Springer EL (1977): Expression of antigenic crossreactivity to RD114 p30 protein in a human fibrosarcoma cell line. Proc Natl Acad Sci USA 74:744–748.

Smith SR, Howell A, Minawa A, Morrison JM (1982): The clinical value of immunohistochemically demonstrable CEA in breast cancer: A possible method of selecting patients for adjuvant/chemotherapy. Br J Cancer 46:757–764.

Snyder HW Jr, Fleissner E (1980): Specificity of human antibodies directed against carbohydrate structures. Proc Natl Acad Sci USA 77:1122–1126.

Sonnendecker EW, DeSouza JJ, Herman AA (1984): Screening for liver metastases from ovarian cancer with serum carcinoembryonic antigen and radionuclide hepatic scintiphotography. Br J Obstet Gynaecol 91:187–192.

Speers WC, Picaso LG, Silverberg SG (1983): Immunohistochemical localization of carcinoembryonic antigen in microglandular hyperplasia and adenocarcinoma of the endocervix. Am J Clin Pathol 79:105–107.

Springer GF (1984): T and Tn, general carcinoma autoantigens. Science 224:1198–1206.

Srivastava BI, Khan SA, Minowada J, Henderson ES, Rakowski I (1980): Terminal deoxynucleotidyl transferase activity and blast cell characteristics in adult acute leukemias. Leuk Res 4:209–215.

Staab HJ, Anderer FA, Brummendorf T, Hornung A, Fischer R (1982a): Prognostic value of preoperative serum CEA level compared to clinical staging: II. Stomach cancer. Br J Cancer 45:718:727.

Staab HJ, Anderer FA, Hornung A, Stumpf E, Fischer R (1982b): Doubling time of circulating CEA and its relation to survival of patients with recurrent colorectal cancer. Br J Cancer 46:773–781.

Stafford MA, Jones OW (1972): The presence of "fetal" thymidine kinase in human tumors. Biochim Biophys Acta 277:439–442.

Starling JJ, Sieg SM, Beckett ML, Schellhammer PF, Ladaga LE, Wright GL (1982): Monoclonal antibodies to human prostate and bladder tumor-associated antigens. Cancer Res 42:3084–3089.

Stea B, Halpern RM, Halpern BC, Smith RA (1981): Urinary excretion levels of unconjugated pterins in cancer patients and normal individuals. Clin Chim Acta 113:231–242.

Steele G Jr, Zamcheck N, Wilson R, Mayer R, Lokich J, Rauz P, Maltz J (1980): Results of CEA-initiated second-look surgery for recurrent colorectal cancer. Am J Surgery 139: 544–548.

Steele G, Ellenberg S, Ramming K, O'Connell M, Moertel C, Lessner H, Bruckner H, Horton J, Schein P, Zamcheck N, Novak J, Holyoke ED (1982): CEA monitoring among patients in multi-institutional adjuvant GI therapy protocols. Ann Surg 196:162–169.

Stefansson K, Wollmann R, Terkovic M (1982): S-100 protein in soft-tissue tumors derived from Schwann cells and melanocytes. Am J Pathol 106:261–268.

Stein H, Bonk A, Tolksdorf G, Lennert K, Rodt H, Gerdes J (1980): Immunohistologic analysis of the organisation of normal lymphoid tissue and non-Hodgkin's lymphomas. J Histochem Cytochem 28:746–760.

Stein H, Tolksdorf G, Lennert K (1981): T-cell lymphomas. A cell origin-related classification on the basis of cytologic, immunologic, and enzyme cytochemical criteria. Pathol Res Pract 171:197–215.

Stein PC, Char DH, Christensen M (1980): Immune complexes in retinoblastoma. Proc Am Assoc Cancer Res 21:373.

Stenman UH, Huhtala ML, Koistinen R, Seppala M (1982): Immunochemical demonstration of an ovarian cancer-associated urinary peptide. Int J Cancer 30:53–57.

Steplewski Z, Koprowski H (1981): Monoclonal antibody defined antigens of human solid tumors. Fed Proc 40:823.

Stramignoni D, Bowen R, Atkinson BF, Schlom J (1983): Differential reactivity of monoclonal antibodies with human colon adenocarcinomas and adenomas. Int J Cancer 31:543–552.

Stuhmiller GM, Seigler HF (1975): Characterization of a chimpanzee antihuman melanoma antiserum. Cancer Res 35:2132–2137.

Stuhmiller GM, Green RW, Seigler HF (1978): Solubilization and partial isolation of human melanoma tumor-associated antigens. J Natl Cancer Inst 61:61–68.

Sullivan AK, Jerry LM, Rowden G, Lewis MG, Pitzele R, Law T, Adams LS, Le Thi H, Shea M (1976): Fetal antigens on the surface of human lymphoid cells. J Exp Med 143:1557–1561.

Summers JL, Coon JS, Ward RM, Falor WH, Miller AW, Weinstein RS (1983): Prognosis in carcinoma of the urinary bladder based upon tissue blood group ABH and Thomsen-Friedenreich antigen status and karyotype of the initial tumor. Cancer Res 43:934–939.

Sundblad G, Edgington TS (1983): Identification of the cytosol form of human mammary tumor glycoprotein (MTGP). Proc Am Assoc Cancer Res 23:921.

Suter L, Sorg C, Mueller R, Johannsen R, Macher E (1975): Membrane associated antigens of human malignant melanoma: I. Internal labeling, detergent solubilization and characterization by homologous antisera and polyacrylamide gel electrophoresis. Z Immunitaetsforsch Exp Klin Immunol 150:318–326.

Syrjanen KJ, Pyrhonen S (1982): Immunoperoxidase demonstration of human papilloma virus (HPV) in dysplastic lesions of the uterine cervix. Arch Gynecol 233:53–61.

Syrjanen K, Vayrynen M, Castren O, Mantyjarvi R, Pyrhonen S, Yliskoski M (1983a): Morphological and immunohistochemical evidence of human papilloma virus (HPV) involvement in the dysplastic lesions of the uterine cervix. Int J Gynaecol Obstet 21: 261–269.

Syrjanen KJ, Pyrhonen S, Syrjanen SM (1983b): Evidence suggesting human papillomavirus (HPV) etiology for the squamous cell papilloma of the paranasal sinus. Arch Geschwulstforsch 53:77–82.

Tabin CJ, Bradley SM, Bargmann CI, Weinberg RA, Papageorge AG, Scolnick EM, Dhar R, Lowy DR, Chang EH (1982): Mechanism of activation of a human oncogene. Nature 300:143–149.

Tabolli S, Valtorta C, Scarda A, D'Erasmo E, Minisola S, Antonelli R, Medori C, Mazzuoli G (1983): Plasma calcitonin and tumors. Tumori 69:227–230.

Tabuchi K, Kirsch WM, Van Buskirk JJ (1978): Immunocytochemical evidence for SV40-related T antigens in two human brain tumours of ependymal origin. Acta Neurochir 43:239–249.

Tai T, Paulson JC, Cahan LD, Irie RF (1983): GM2 ganglioside as human tumor antigen (OFA-I-1). Proc Am Assoc Cancer Res 23:892.

Takahashi A, Yachi A, Anzai T, Wada T (1967): Presence of a unique serum protein in sera obtained from patients with neoplastic diseases and in embryonic and neonatal sera. Clin Chim Acta 17:5–12.

Takahashi K, Isobe T, Ohtsuki Y, Sonobe H, Takeda I and Akagi T (1984): Immunohistochemical localization and distribution of S-100 proteins in the human lymphoreticular system. Am J Pathol 116:497–503.

Takeuchi T, Tujiki H, Kameya T (1981): Characterization of amylases produced by tumors. Clin Chem 27:556–559.

Tal C, Halperin M (1970): Presence of serologically distinct protein in serum of cancer patients and pregnant women. Israel J Med Sci 6:708–716.

Talerman A, Haije WG, Baggerman L (1971): Alpha-1 antitrypsin (AAT) and alphafetoprotein (AFP) in sera of patients with germ-cell neoplasms: Value as tumour markers in patients with endodermal sinus tumour (yolk sac tumour). Int J Cancer 19:741–746.

Tan MH, Shimano T, Chu TM (1981): Differential localization of human pancreas cancer-associated antigen and carcinoembryonic antigen in homologous pancreatic tumoral xenograft. J Natl Cancer Inst 67:563–569.

Tanaka F, Amino N, Hayashi C, Miyai K, Kumahara Y (1976): Abnormal serum lactate dehydrogenase isoenzyme in a case of laryngeal carcinoma and thyrotoxicosis. Clin Chim Acta 68:235–240.

Taniguchi N, Yokosawa N, Narita M, Mitsuyama T, Makita A (1981): Expression of Frossman antigen synthesis and degradation in human lung cancer. J Natl Cancer Inst 67: 577–583.

Tataryn DN, MacFarlane JK, Thomson DM (1978) Leukocyte adherence inhibition for detecting specific tumor immunity in early pancreatic cancer. Lancet 1:1020–1022.

Tatsuta M, Yamamoto R, Yamamura H, Okuda S, Tamura H (1983): Cytologic examination and CEA measurement in aspirated pancreatic material collected by percutaneous fine-needle aspiration biopsy under ultrasonic guidance for the diagnosis of pancreatic carcinoma. Cancer 52:693–698.

Taub RN, Roncari DA, Baker MA (1978): Isolation and partial characterization of radioiodinated myeloblastic leukemia-associated cell surface antigen. Cancer Res 38:4624–4629.

Taylor CM, Yeoman LC, Busch FN, Busch H (1980): Analysis of nuclear and cytoplasmic antigens in GW-39 colon tumor cells by isoelectric focusing and crossed immunoelectrophoresis. Proc Am Assoc Cancer Res 21:246.

Teichmann B, Vogt R (1974): Isolation of tumor localizing antibodies by immunosorbents. III. Isolation of heterologous antibodies for human cervical carcinoma and renal carcinoma. Arch Geschwulstforsch. 43:145–156.

Teramato YA, Mariani R, Wunderlich D, Schlom J (1982): The immunohistochemical reactivity of a human monoclonal antibody with tissue sections of human mammary tumors. Cancer 50:241–249.

Terui S, (1984): Clinical evaluation of thyroxine-binding globulin (TBG) as a marker of liver tumors. Eur J Nucl Med 9:121–124.

Than GN, Csaba IF, Szabo DG, Bognar ZJ, Arany A, Bohn H (1983): Levels of placenta-specific tissue protein 12(PP12) in serum during normal pregnancy and in patients with trophoblastic tumour. Arch Gynecol 234:39–46.

Thomas BS, Bulbrook RD, Hayward JL, Millis RR (1982): Urinary androgen metabolites and recurrence rates in early breast cancer. Eur J Clin Oncol 18:447–451.

Thomas JA, Janossy G (1982): Phenotypic analysis of cells in cutaneous lymphoma—An immunohistologic study. In Goos M, Christophus E (eds): "Lymphoproliferative Diseases of the Skin." Berlin: Springer-Verlag, pp 128–136.

Thompson CH, Jones SL, Pihl E, McKenzie IF (1983a): Monoclonal antibodies to human colon and colorectal carcinoma. Br J Cancer 47:595–605.

Thompson CH, Jones SL, Whitehead RH, McKenzie IF (1983b): A human breast tissue-associated antigen detected by monoclonal antibody. J Natl Cancer Inst 70:409–419.

Thompson RJ, Rubery ED, Jones HM (1980): Radioimmunoassay of serum creatine kinase-BB as a tumour marker in breast cancer. Lancet 2:673–675.

Thomson DM, Tataryn DN, Weatherhead JC, Friedlander P, Rauch J, Schwartz R, Gold P, Shuster J (1980): A human colon tumour antigen associated with β-microglobulin and isolated from solid tumour, serum and urine is unrelated to carcinoembryonic antigen. Eur J Cancer 16:547–551.

Thomson DMP, Rauch JE, Weatherhead JC, Friedlander P, O'Connor R, Grosser N, Shuster J, Gold P (1978): Isolation of human tumour-specific antigens associated with β_2-microglobulin. J Cancer 37:753–755.

Thorne HJ, Jose DG, Adams FC, Coelen RJ, Whitehead RH, Klugg G (1982): Children's brain tumour cells produce RNA particles with incomplete retrovirus characteristics. Oncology 39:156–162.

Thorpe WP, Rosenberg SA (1977): Expression of fetal antigens by normal human adult skin cells and human sarcoma cells in tissue culture: Implications for studies in human tumor immunology. Proc Am Assoc Cancer Res 18:206.

Thorpe WP, Rosenberg SA (1978): Identification of tumor specific antigens on human osteogenic sarcoma. Proc Am Assoc Cancer Res 19:107.

Tilgen W, Hellström I, Engstner M, Garrigues HJ, Riehl R, Hellström KE (1983): Localization of melanoma-associated antigen p97 in cultured human melanoma, as visualized by light and electron microscopy. J Invest Dermatol 80:459–463.

Tobinani K, Nagai M, Setoya T, Shibata T, Minato K, Shimoyama M (1983): Anti-ATLA (Antibody to adult T-cell leukemia virus-associated antigen), highly positive on OKTH-positive mature T-cell malignancies. Jpn J Clin Oncol 12:237–244.

Tomana M, Niedermeier W, Mukherjee D (1981a): Antibodies to MMTV-related antigen in breast cancer patients of different ages. Cancer Immuno Immunother 11:59–61.

Tomana M, Kajdos AH, Niedermeier W, Durkin WJ, Mestecky J (1981b): Antibodies to mouse mammary tumor virus-related antigen in sera of patients with breast carcinoma. Cancer 47:2696–2703.

Tomoda H, Furusawa M, Seo Y, Matsukuchi T, Miyazaka M, Kanashima R (1982): Measurement of serum ferritin in various digestive diseases by reversed passive hemagglutination using anti-human placental ferritin antiserum. Jpn J Clin Oncol 12:9–16.

Tourine R, Deschamps O (1982): Carcinoembryonic antigen (CEA) levels in pleural effusions associated with bronchogenic carcinoma, extra-thoracic malignancies, and benign diseases. Eur J Respir Dis 63:112.

Toya D, Sawabu N, Ozaki K, Wakabayashi T, Nakagen M, Hattori N (1983): Purification of gamma-glutamyltranspeptidase (gamma-GTP) from human hepatocellular carcinoma (HCC) and comparison of gamma-GTP with the enzyme from human kidney. Ann NY Acad Sci 417:86–96.

Toyama S (1983): Detection of human osteosarcoma-associated antigens by monoclonal antibodies. Gan T Kagaku Ryoho 10:1013–1020.

Tracey KJ, O'Brien MJ, Williams LF, Klibaner M, George PK, Saravis CA, Zamchek N (1984): Signet ring carcinoma of the pancreas, a rare variant with very high CEA values. Immunohistologic comparison with adenocarcinoma. Dig Dis Sci 29:573–576.

Tränhardt H, Zintl F, Milleck J, Plenert W (1978): Fötale Antigene auf Leukämiezellen. Arch Geschwulstforsch 48:750–755.

Trehan S, Rao N, Shetty PA, Noronha JM (1982): Urinary 6-hydroxymethylpterin levels accurately monitor response to chemotherapy in acute myeloblastic leukemia. Cancer 50:114–117.

Trouillas P (1971): Carcino-fetal antigen in glial tumours. Lancet 2:552.

Tsang KT, Singh I, Fudenberg HH (1980): Isolation of tumor-specific antibody from patients with human osteosarcoma. Fed Proc 39:1144.

Tsang KY, Pan JF, Fudenberg HH (1984): Production of antibody to human osteosarcoma-associated antigens by continuous human lymphoblastoid cell lines. Immunol Lett 7:267–272.

Tsang PH, Holland JF, Bekesi JG (1982): Specificity of tumor antigen recognition by T-lymphocytes in the leukocyte adherence inhibition (LAI) assay in patients with breast cancer. J Clin Lab Immunol 9:151–157.

Tsokos M, Linnoila RI, Chandra RS, Triche TJ (1984): Neuron-specific enolase in the diagnosis of neuroblastoma and other small, round-cell tumors in children. Hum Pathol 15:575–584.

Tsou KC, Lo KW, Witzleben CL, Suganuma T (1982): An immunohistochemical 5′-nucleotide phosphodiesterase method for the diagnosis of liver cancer in human liver biopsy. Proc Am Assoc Cancer Res 23:67.

Tsou KC, Lo KW, Rosato EF, Yuk A, Enterline, H, Schwegman C (1982a): Evaluation of 5′-nucleotide phosphodiesterase isoenzyme-V as a predictor of liver metastatis in breast cancer patients. Cancer 50:191–196.

Tsuchida Y, Hasegawa H (1983): The diagnostic value of alpha-fetoprotein in infants and children with teratomas: A questionnaire survey in Japan. J Pediatr Surg 18:152–155.

Tsuchiya T, Noda T, Niyamoto T, Taniguchi H (1980): Alpha-1-antitrypsin in tumors of the pancreas. Nippon Rinsho 38:146–151.

Tsujimoto Y, Yunis J, Onorato-Showe L, Erikson J, Nowell PC, Croce CM (1984): Molecular cloning of the chromosomal breakpoint of B-cell lymphomas and leukemias with the t (11;14) chromosome translocation. Science 224:1403–1406.

Tsukuda M, Sawaki S, Yanoma S, Yoshimura N, Takei M, Tekada M, Sudo K, Suzuki K, Kawamura A (1980): Nasopharyngeal carcinoma membrane soluble antigen. Jpn J Exp Med 50:79–84.

Tsutsumi Y, Nagura H, Watanabe K (1984): Immunohistochemical observations of carcinoembryonic antigen (CEA) and CEA-related substances in normal and neoplastic pancreas. Am J Clin Pathol 82:535–542.

Turner GA, Ellis RD, Guthrie D, Latner AL, Ross WM, Skillen AW (1982): Cyclic GMP in urine to monitor the response of ovarian cancer to therapy. Br J Obstet Gynaecol 89: 760–764.

Udayachander M, Meenakshi A, Ansamma J, Muthiah R (1983): Lymphoma-associated antigen (LAA): Isolation, characterization and clinical evaluation. Br J Cancer 48: 717–725.

Ueda R (1983): Analysis of cell surface antigen of kidney cancer by autologous sera and monoclonal antibodies. Gan To Kagaku 10:1542–1549.

Ueda R, Morrissey D, Ogata SI, Finstad C, Whitmore WF, Lloyd KO, Oettgen HF, Old LJ (1981): Human renal cancer cell surface antigens defined by mouse monoclonal antibodies. Proc Am Assoc Cancer Res 22:304.

Ueda S, Tsubura A, Izumi H, Sadaki M, Morii S (1983): Immunohistochemical studies on carcinoembryonic antigen in adenocarcinomas of the uterus. Acta Pathol Jpn 33:59–69.

Ulich TR, Yang K, Wen DR, Cochran AJ, Lewin KJ (1982): S-100-like immunoreactivity in neuroendocrine tumors. Gastroenterology 82:1200.

Utsunomiya Matsumoto M, Nishioka K, Iwahashi M, Hanada S, Nomura K, Hashimoto S, Yunoki K (1983): A report of a case of T-cell-derived chronic lymphocytic leukemia with antibodies to adult T-cell leukemia-associated antigens. Jpn J Clin Oncol 13:291–299,

Vaczi L, Toth FD (1980): Studies of antigens of C-type primate viruses and antibodies to them in patients with myeloid leukemia and potentially preleukemic hematological disorders. Arch Geschwulstforsch 50:769–777.

Vaitukaitis JL, Ross GT, Braunstein GD, Rayford PL (1976): Gonadotropins and their subunits: Basic and clinical studies. Recent Prog Hormone Res 32:289–331.

Van Alstyne D (1977): Hemagglutination as an alternate technique for the detection of melanoma-specific cytoplasmic antigens. Am J Clin Pathol 68:24–48.

Van Cangh PJ, Opsomer R, De Nayer P (1982) Serum prostatic acid phosphatase determination in prostatic disease: A critical comparison of an emzymatic and a radioimmunologic assay. J Urol 128:1212–1215.

Van Kley H, Cramer S, Bruns DE (1981): Serous ovarian neoplastic amylase (SONA): A potentially useful marker for serous ovarian tumors. Cancer 48:1444–1449.

Varki NM, Reisfeld RA, Walker LE (1984): Antigens associated with human lung adenocarcinoma defined by monoclonal antibodies. Cancer Res 44:681–687.

Vecchio FM, Fabiano A, Ghirlanda G, Manna R, Massi G (1984): Fibrolamellar carcinoma of the liver: The malignant counterpart of focal nodular hyperplasia with oncocytic change. Am J Clin Pathol 81:521–525.

Vennegoor C, Jonker A, Van Smeerdi D, Van Es A, Rumke P (1977): Specificity of a monkey antiserum for a melanoma cell line IPC-48. Protides Biol Fluid Proc Colloq 25:731–734.

Vesce F, Biondi C (1983): Alpha-L-fucosidase activity in endometrial cervical and ovarian cancer. Eur J Gynaecol Oncol 4:135–138.

Viza D, Phillips J (1975): Identification of an antigen associated with malignant melanoma. Int J Cancer 16:312–317.

Viza D, Davies DAL, Harris R (1970): Solubilization and partial purification of human leukemia specific antigens. Nature 227:1249–1251.

Viza D, Louvier M, Phillips J, Boucheix C, Guerin RA (1975): Solubilization of an antigen associated with certain bronchial tumours. Eur J Cancer 11:765–770.

Von Eyben FE (1983): Lactate dehydrogenase and its isoenzymes in testicular germ cell tumors: An overview. Oncodev Biol Med 4:395–414.

Waalkes TP, Abeloff MD, Ettinger DS, Woo KB, Gehrke CW, Kuo KC, Borek E (1982): Modified ribonucleosides as biological markers for patients with small cell carcinoma of the lung. Eur J Cancer Clin Oncol 18:1267–1274.

Waalkes TP, Abeloff MD, Ettinger DS, Woo KB, Koo KC, Gehrke CW (1983): Serum protein-bound carbohydrates and small cell carcinoma of the lung. Correlations with extent of disease, tumor burden survival, and clinical response categories. Cancer 52:131–139.

Wada T, Anzai T, Yachi A, Takahashi A, Sakamoto S-I (1970): Incidences of three different fetal proteins in sera of patients with primary hepatoma. Protides Biol Fluids Proc Colloq 18:221–226.

Waghe M, Kumar S (1977): Demonstration of a Wilms' tumour associated antigen using xenogenic antiserum (preliminary communication). Eur J Cancer 13:993–998.

Wagner W, Husemann B, Becker H, Groitl H, Koerfgen HP, Hammerschmidt M (1982): Tissue polypeptide antigen—A new tumour marker? Aust NZ Surg 52:41–43.

Wahlstrom T, Linder E, Saksela E, Westermark B (1974): Tumor-specific membrane antigens in established cell lines from gliomas. Cancer 34:274–279.

Wahren B, Nilsson B, Zimmerman R (1982): Urinary CEA for prediction of survival time and recurrence in bladder cancer. Cancer 50:139–145.

Waldmann TA, McIntire KR (1974): The use of radioimmunoassay for alpha-fetoprotein in the diagnosis of malignancy. Cancer 34:1510–1515.

Walker C, Gray BN (1983): Acute-phase reactant proteins and carcinoembryonic antigen in cancer of the colon and rectum. Cancer 52:150–154.

Walker PD, Karnik S, deKernion JB, Pramberg JC (1984): Cell surface blood group antigens in prostatic carcinoma. Am J Clin Pathol 81:503–506.

Wallach SR, Royston I, Taetle R, Wohl H, Deftos LJ (1981): Plasma calcitonin as a marker of disease activity in patients with small cell carcinoma of the lung. J Clin Endocrinol Metab 53:602–606.

Walts AE, Said JW, Shintaku IP, Sassoon AF, Banks-Schlegel S (1984): Keratins of different molecular weight in exfoliated mesothelial and adenocarcinoma cells—an aid to cell identification. Am J Clin Pathol 81:442–446.

Wang DY, Knyba RE, Bulbrook RD, Millis RR, Hayward JL (1984): Serum carcinoembryonic antigen in the diagnosis and prognosis of women with breast cancer. Eur J Cancer Clin Oncol 20:25–31.

Wang MC, Valenzuela L, Murphy GP, Chu TM (1977): Tissue specific and tumor specific antigens in human prostate. Fed Proc 36:1254.

Warshaw AL, Lee KH, Wood WC, Cohen AM, (1980): Sensitivity and specificity of serum ribonuclease in the diagnosis of pancreatic cancer. Am J Surg 139:27–32.

Watanabe T (1980): Pregnancy-associated alpha-2-glycoprotein and carcinoembryonic antigen in the sera of patients with lung cancer. Iwate Igaku Zasshi 32:519–530.

Watanabe A, Nagshima H (1981): Altered dynamics of alpha-fetoprotein production following pyridoxine and adenosine 5′-triphosphate administration to cirrhotic patients with or without primary hepatomas and to liver-injured hepatoma-bearing rats. Oncodev Biol Med 2:313–321.

Watson RD, Smith AG, Levy JG (1975): The detection by immunodiffusion of tumour associated antigenic components in extracts of human bronchogenic carcinoma. Br J Cancer 32:300–309.

Weikang S, Yanling L, Min Y, Zhen Y (1977): Membrane-associated embryonic antigen in human hepato-cellular carcinoma cells. Acta Zool Sin 23:344.

Weickmann JL, Olson EM, Glitz DG (1984): Immunological assay of pancreatic ribonuclease in serum as an indicator of pancreatic cancer. Cancer Res 44:1682–1687.

Weiss AF, Portmann R, Fischer H, Simon J, Zang KA (1975): Simian virus 40-related antigens in three human meningiomas with defined chromosome loss. Proc Natl Acad Sci USA 72:609–613.

Weiss AF, Zang KD, Birkmayer GD, Miller F (1976): SV40 related Papova-viruses in human meningiomas. Acta Neuropathol 34:171–174.

Weiss MA, Michel JG, Pesce AJ, DiPersio L (1981): Heterogeneity of $\beta,\epsilon,\tau,\alpha,\eta_2$-microglobulin in human breast carcinoma. Lab Invest 45:46–57.

Whitson ME, Lozzio CB, Lozzio BB, Wust CJ, Sonoda T, Avery B (1976): Cytotoxicity of antisera to a myelogenous leukemia cell line with the Philadelphia chromosome. J Natl Cancer Inst 56:903–907.

Wick MR, Scheithauer BW, Kovacs K (1983): Neuron-specific enolase in neuroendocrine tumors of the thymus, bronchus, and skin. Am J Clin Pathol 79:703–707.

Wiels J, Fellous M, Lenoir G, Tursz T (1982): A monoclonal antibody defining a Burkitt lymphoma associated antigen. Protides Biol Fluid Proc Colloq 29:899–902.

Wikstrand CJ, Bigner DD (1979): Surface antigens of human glioma cells shared with normal adult and fetal brain. Cancer Res 39:3235–3243.

Wikstrand CJ, Bigner DD (1982): Expression of human fetal brain antigens by human tumors of neuroectodermal origin as defined by monoclonal antibodies. Cancer Res 42:267–275.

Wikstrand CJ, Bigner SH, Bigner DD (1984): Characterization of three restricted specificity monoclonal antibodies raised against the human glioma cell line D-54 MG. J Neuroimmunol 6:169–186.

Wikstrand CJ, Mahaley MS, Bigner DD (1977): Surface antigenic characteristics of human glial brain tumor cells. Cancer Res 37:4267–4275.

Wikstrand CJ, Bourdon MA, Pegram CN, Bigner DD (1982): Human fetal brain antigen expression common to tumors of neuroectodermal tissue origin. J Neuroimmunol 3:43–62.

Wikstrand SJ, Pegram CN, Bourdon MA (1981): Expression of human fetal brain antigens (FBA) by human glioblastoma (HGL) cells as defined by monoclonal antibodies. Proc Am Assoc Cancer Res 22:304.

Wiley EL, Mendelsohn G, Droller MJ, Eggleston JC (1982): Immunoperoxidase detection of carcinoembryonic antigen and blood group substances in papillary transitional cell carcinoma of the bladder. J Urol 128:276–280.

Winkel P, Bentzon MW, Statland BE, Mouridsen H, Sheike O (1982): Predicting recurrence in patients with breast cancer from cumulative laboratory results: A new technique for the application of time series analysis. Clin Chem 28:2057–2067.

Winters WD, Rich JR (1975): Human meningioma antigens. Int J Cancer 15:815–822.

Wolf A, Mickschc M, Bauer H (1981): An improved antigenic marker of human lung carcinomas and its use in radioimmunoassays. Br J Cancer 43:267–275.

Woodbury RG, Brown JP, Yeh MY, Hellström I, Hellström KE (1980): Identification of a cell surface protein, P97, in human melanomas and certain other neoplasms. Proc Natl Acad Sci 77:2183–2187.

Wright GL, Schellhammer PF, Faulconer RL (1977): Isolation of a soluble tumor-associated antigen from human renal cell carcinoma by gradient acrylamide gel electrophoresis. Cancer Res 37:4228–4232.

Wright GL, Schellhammer PF, Rosato FE, Faulconer RJ (1978): Detection of tumor-associated antigen in soluble extracts of urogenital tumors. Proc Am Assoc Cancer Res 19:13.

Wright GL Jr, Starling JJ, Sieg SM (1981): Monoclonal antibodies to tumor-associated antigens in human prostate and bladder cancer. Fed Proc 40:995.

Wurz H, Luben G, Bohn H (1983): Serum levels of placental protein 10 (PP10) in women with breast cancer and genital carcinoma and in healthy male and female subjects. Arch Gynecol 233:267–274.

Yachi A, Matsumura Y, Carpenter CM, Hyde L (1968): Immunochemical studies of human lung cancer antigens soluble in 50% saturated ammonium sulfate. J Natl Cancer Inst 40:663–682.

Yam LT, Janekila AJ, Li CY, Lam WK (1981): Presence of "prostatic" acid phosphatase in human neutrophils. Invest Urol 19:34–38.

Yamamoto N (1983): Biology of adult T-cell leukemia virus. Gan To Kagaku Ryoho 10:674–679.

Yamamoto N, Chosa T, Koyanagi Y, Tochikura T, Schneider J, Hinuma Y (1984): Binding of adult T-cell leukemia virus to various hematopoietic cells. Cancer Lett 21:261–268.

Yu GSM, Kadish AS, Johnson AD, Marcus DM (1980): Breast carcinoma-associated antigen. An immunocytochemical study. Am J Clin Pathol 74:453–456.

Zarabi MC, Rupani M (1984): Human chorionic gonadotropin-secreting pure dysgerminoma. Hum Pathol 15:589–592.

Zeltzer PM, Marangos PJ, Parma AM, Sather H, Dalton A, Hammond D, Siegel SE, Seeger RC (1983): Raised neuron-specific enolase in serum of children with metastatic neuroblastoma. A report from the children's cancer study group. Lancet 2:361–363.

Zenner HP (1981): Monoclonal antibodies against surface antigens of laryngeal carcinoma cells. Arch Otorhinolaryngol 233:161–172.

Zimmerman R, Wahren B (1976): Characterization of carcinoembryonic antigen (CEA) from bladder carcinomas. Third International Symposium on Detection and Prevention of Cancer (Meeting Abstract), p 257.

Index